I Wa...
be Healed

JUDITH COLLINS is a renowned healer, author and edu-
cator, and is recognised as Australia's leading authority on
the human aura. Judith founded the Earthkeepers Healing
Sanctuary in NSW where she treats many chronically ill
patients and people seeking insight into their personal well-
being. In 1983 Judith was awarded the prestigious *Advance
Australia Award*. In the 1988 Bicentennial celebrations she was
recognised as one of Australia's unsung heroines and her
life's service to the community was documented. Judith
appears regularly on television and radio and she writes for a
number of magazines and newspapers. She also lectures and
holds workshops at the *Mind, Body and Spirit Festival* around
Australia, and internationally.

I dedicate this book to the Divine Spirit which entered my life in
order that I may serve others;
and to Max Cuthbert, John Livingstone, Donna Maberly
and Mervyn Wale
who taught me so much on their journey to death.

I Want to be Healed

Judith Collins

Lothian
BOOKS

Other titles by this author

Affirmations for Life
How to See and Read the Human Aura
Companion Gardening in Australia

Thomas C. Lothian Pty Ltd
11 Munro Street, Port Melbourne, Victoria 3207

National Library of Australia
Cataloguing-in-Publication data:

Collins, Judith (Judith Louise).

  I want to be healed.

  ISBN 0 85091 907 X.

  1. Healing. I. Title.

615.852

Cover and text design by Stanley Wong
Typeset by Figment
Printed by Griffin Press Pty Ltd
Photographs by Frank Leitner

The article on page 1 by Peter Tute appears courtesy of the *Macarthur Chronicle* and
is printed with the permission of Cumberland Newspaper Group.
The poem on page 24, 'The Little Shoes that Died' from *Selected Poems* by Mary
Gilmore, appears courtesy of ETT Imprint, Sydney, 1998.

CONTENTS

Acknowledgements

This book would not have been possible without my sharing of the healing experience with all my clients. I thank you for enriching my life.

I would especially like to acknowledge and thank those who contributed to this book: my husband Paul for his creative artwork which helps to enhance my message, my secretary Sharon Webber for her tireless support, my mother for her faith, and all those who shared their healing testimony with readers.

Judith Collins

1

HOW I CAME TO HEAL

In June 1994, Camden resident Shawna McCoy was gravely ill with thyroid cancer. Diagnosed as a terminal illness, the disease had defeated the best efforts of surgeons. Judith Collins gave her a second chance at life. After a number of visits to Judith at Earthkeepers Healing Sanctuary at Thirlmere, Shawna's cancer was cured — a miracle perhaps but just another day's work for Judith.

Despite the fact that a number of people are prepared to testify to her powers, this happy-go-lucky healer does not see herself as a miracle worker. Indeed, her casual manner and habit of quoting lines from *Monty Python* films make it difficult to hail her as a messianic figure, which suits her just fine.

Judith does not question her abilities to try to explain how they work. 'This power is not from me, it's through me — it works because it is Divine' she said. 'Anything meant to be cured will be cured.' This can be frustrating for anyone trying to understand spiritual healing but sceptics do not concern Judith. 'It works on sceptics too. It converts them — I love that.'

She is not operating on the fringes of naturopathy either. Qualified doctors refer patients to her and she has an ever-growing clientele around Australia and the world.

Peter Tute, *The Chronical,* May 1995

WHEN PEOPLE ask me how I discovered my healing powers I promptly recall an event which occurred while I was travelling from work to my home some years ago. The traffic was banked up for miles, or so it seemed. A deep yet gentle masculine voice echoed through the car saying, 'Go forth and put your left hand on the little boy's chest and your right hand on his head'. I repeatedly looked around to see who could be saying this but saw no one. The voice persisted in an urgent, beckoning tone. A deep and wonderful drifting silence followed but was shattered abruptly by a piercing female voice asking, 'What's wrong with him?'. I opened my eyes and found myself kneeling, with my hands placed exactly in the position which the male voice had instructed. I panicked. Crowds of people had gathered around the little boy. The woman pushed me aside while declaring her nursing credentials. Suddenly I realised that I was 200 metres from my car.

A numbness swept over me. I couldn't speak. My husband Paul recalls my face as being a peaceful, ghostly white. Three hours passed before I fully regained my faculties of hearing and speaking. I told him of my experience. I could only remember hearing the initial masculine voice. I don't recall leaving the car nor knowing that an injured child was the cause of the traffic jam, let alone thinking I could place my hands on him to bring about pain relief or heal his wounds.

For several months I avoided travelling alone in the hope that I would prevent the loss of power over my own body. A year passed. My sister-in-law invited me to accompany her to an introductory seminar on homoeopathy. The evening proceeded well until question time. I felt a disturbing tug at the back of my head but when I looked no one was there. I became agitated and the instructor noticed. After dismissing the class she approached me, asking what was the matter. I whimpered as I tried to explain the ordeal. Although reluctant at first, I soon discovered how good it felt to talk to someone. She was compassionate and caring, holding me as a mother comforts a frightened infant. She suggested that someone was trying to contact me from the other side. I ignorantly asked 'the other side of what?'. A long and careful explanation of the Spirit realm unfolded. Escorting me to the car, she placed a folded piece of paper into my hand. It read 'David, Clairvoyant, telephone...'. And before I set off, she had me promise to contact him.

Upon arriving home I propped the message against the mirror on my dressing table in order to remind me to make an appointment. Each day I stared at it. Two months had passed before I questioned myself as to why I had not followed up this contact. What do I want with a so-called clairvoyant, I argued? My thoughts were haunted by concepts I had encountered in my Christian childhood such as devil worship and evil people. After assuring myself that I was of good intent, that at all times I tried to be fair and that I never sought to harm anyone, I reached the conclusion that I was not possessed nor about to be. So, I confirmed an appointment to consult with David.

My husband and I sat parked outside David's house for a full fifteen minutes while my mind summoned the courage to go through with it. A polite young man in his late twenties, came to the door and invited me in. He wore peace and gentleness like a cloak. I felt safe.

Sitting opposite each other he took my hand and said: 'You have been born with the gift of second sight and it has manifested itself as "auric vision" — the ability to see and read the human energy field. You have a special purpose and are surrounded by evolved spirits who will guide and help you. Your life will become so busy that a diary and a secretary will prove essential to organise your schedule and cope with the public demand on your time. You will be called on to write several books and magazine articles, as well as appear on both radio and television'. He paused, staring above and around my head. 'You are also surrounded by dozens of spirits of children, who will make themselves known to you in the fullness of time.'

By this stage I was flabbergasted and appreciative that the session was being recorded. Curiously, David repeatedly insisted that I would be tutored not on Earth but in heaven.

I immediately drew the conclusion that he was attempting to tell me that I would die at a young age. He quickly allayed my fears and added one last message: 'You have only half the key and will therefore only know half the success. But there is one who is associated with horses who will fully turn the key to open many doors to you. When this occurs, you will know you have reached the pinnacle of success'.

Night after night my husband and I listened to the tape, trying to analyse the message. We challenged its credibility and tried to evaluate the experience. David had told me about my grandmother, my parents and many childhood experiences I knew to be accurate and I felt confident that he was truly gifted. It was just his final comment which unsettled me: 'I am in awe of your gifts and so too will be people all over the world'.

Unable to fathom the clairvoyant session I decided to let life unfold as I felt that the whole episode had already taken up too much of my time. I was rather complacent until a few weeks later. A woman in her late thirties appeared on my doorstep asking for healing. I was puzzled and explained that she was asking the wrong person. Crying and pleading with me to heal her of infertility she emotionally manoeuvred her way into my house. We sat and talked for a while. Then to make her happy I placed my left hand on the back of her head. She closed her eyes and looked as if something was about to happen. Within moments a bright white light changed the atmosphere of the room and my hands began to tingle. A male voice echoed in the distance, 'Put your right hand over her forehead and hold until you feel my contribution'.

As I moved my hand to follow the instruction I felt a warm flow of air at the tips of my fingers and saw gold sparks of light, shimmering like sparklers on cracker night. In a moment of curiosity I asked 'Who are you?'. Suddenly I became cocooned in a web of wholeness. Then the voice replied, 'I am known by many as Martin de Porres' (a Christian saint and healer). As he spoke I felt my fear of the unknown swept away by the flow of love in the room. I asked if he was healing through me. He explained that he was a

messenger for a Divine source, known to Christians as the
Holy Spirit. He referred me to a catholic mass being celebrated by a visiting priest with healing powers. Although not
keen on returning to the clutches of the church I was nonethe-
less intrigued.

Some time later the woman returned to tell me that she was
pregnant and how she had spread the news of my healing
power. The public began to beat a path to my door — one per
day, three per day, then slowly more and more each day.

A client also heard of the visiting priest. He asked if
I would accompany him. I was intrigued with how St Martin
was guaranteeing my attendance. The Lord works in mysterious ways.

The evening was bitterly cold. The church reeked of des-
peration and devotion — peculiar bedfellows I thought. All
manner of people suffering physical and psychological disease and seeking a miracle cure, were present. The priest
moved through his duties with gracious ease. Just moments
before commencing healing by the laying on of hands he said
this: 'I would like to call your attention and ask you to reflect
on what St Paul has to tell us:

> There is a variety of gifts but always the same Spirit; there are
> all sorts of service to be done, but always to the same Lord;
> working in all sorts of different ways in different people, it is
> the same God who is working in all of them. The particular
> way in which the Spirit is given to each person is for a good
> purpose. One may have the gift of preaching with wisdom
> given him by the Spirit; another the gift of faith by the same
> Spirit; another again the gift of healing, through this one
> Spirit; one, the power of miracles; another, prophecy; another
> the gift of recognising spirits; another the gift of tongues and
> another the ability to interpret them; all these are the work of
> one and the same Spirit, who distributes different gifts to dif-
> ferent people just as he chooses.'

1 Cor. 12:4–11

There it was, my message: authority to heal. It was as
though I was being encouraged and comforted at the same
time. I felt a magnetic pull towards the altar. As I stood tall
and still, tears welled in my eyes — not from fear nor from

pain. I couldn't identify their source but tried to control them all the same. Thoughts wrestled with my conscience as the priest approached me.

Opening my mind to the Divine, I took a deep breath to relax. As the priest placed his right hand on my head and prayed, a bolt of what felt like electricity shot through my skull to my feet and then out of my forehead. He looked into my eyes and smiled. As he moved along the row to serve others he frequently stared back at me in wonder. My husband, sister-in-law and brother who had accompanied me, noticed this too. What did he know or recognise, they thought.

On the way home St Martin spoke to me and explained that the priest had been spiritually directed to repeat an invocation to facilitate my initiation to healing in the service of the Spirit. Filled with awe, I hardly slept a wink that night. A new journey had begun.

Enthusiastically my husband converted two rooms in a building on our property to accommodate my new found vocation and I began to work as a healer. No advertising was necessary. People came by word of mouth. Initially they came from the local region and then from further afield, some hundreds and hundreds of miles away from my new clinic. As my work flourished more rooms were constructed and a secretary was employed just as David the clairvoyant had predicted.

One warm March day I received a telephone call from a local naturopath asking if I could treat her friend that afternoon. As it so happened one appointment was free. The urgency was not her illness but the fact that she was booked on a return flight home to Western Australia that afternoon. Then as fate declared its upper hand, an hour later I received a call from a natural health practitioner in Western Australia who was enquiring if I ever worked in Perth. Apparently I had treated her cousin who lived in New South Wales. Then, as if part of a conspiracy, the next person I treated in my clinic announced that he was visiting relatives and wondered if I could ever visit his home base, Perth. By the end of the day I realised that Perth was coming into my life. And I was proved right.

A subsequent phone call from my 'urgent' Perth lady was enticing. She had used her network to ensure enough appointments to cover my expenses and tentatively booked a venue for me to give a public address.

The flight was uneventful, presenting an opportunity to relax and contemplate acceptance of the information I was about to share with my audience. As the crowd gathered and found their seats, the auras of two people stood out: Ruth Carlsson, a woman whose aura displayed a combination of healing and counselling coupled with a wonderful array of life-experience; and Leo Nester, a small statue of a man, whose aura showed he was fraught with anxiety in search of a cure for his wife's cancer. The sparks of light which shone from his fingers enticed me to label him 'nimble fingers'. He had studied Bowen therapy plus a few other healing modalities. Ruth explained how she had been widowed at a young age and had worked long and hard to raise three children. She chose the healing profession because of an eagerness to help people.

During the course of the day I paid special attention to their learning as I felt confident that in the future I would refer my clients to both of them.

On my second trip to Perth an allergy to cigarette smoke rendered me almost voiceless. In order to complete my lecture tour I called upon Ruth to act as a vehicle for healing me. Following my instructions she placed her hands over my nasal passage and jaw line, relaxed and closed her eyes. I called forth to the Spirit realm in my mind and asked for Divine intervention. The temperature of the room increased, a feeling I had come to know as an indication of Spirit presence. A sensation of very hot pins and needles spread from my brow to my jaw. I wondered if this was what acupuncture felt like. The hotter the healing became, the deeper my trance-like state. Feeling what I thought to be a cool fan blowing across my face I returned to the reality of consciousness.

Ruth was speechless so I gave her some space to gather her thoughts. Although she looked pale in colour, she appeared younger in years. On gaining her composure Ruth reported being filled with love as a man stepped inside her body causing her to expand in shape, size and dimension. Her clearest memory was of his hands — strong, yet gentle. St Martin had come to my rescue.

As the tour of Western Australia drew to a close St Martin suggested he stay with Ruth for a while to develop her healing skills. I returned to an ever-busy clinic, more attuned and more aware of the holiness of the healing.

In this first year basic healing skills were shown to me by the Spirit realm mostly while working on clients and at other times through voices and visions. I learnt to open myself to the Divine source of love and gain knowledge of methods of approach to the healing and soothing of a variety of ailments such as infertility, cancer, heart disease, multiple sclerosis, chronic fatigue and burns. It was a trying period because my beliefs were repeatedly challenged and remoulded in preparation for the role my life now plays.

Healing has been a highlight in my life. It has been shaped and reshaped by the believers and the non-believers. Even a member of the Australian Sceptics Inc. sought to challenge my skills by masquerading as a client. The whole encounter prompted me to re-evaluate my beliefs and experiences, thus reinforcing my commitment to serve the community in whatever way I'm called.

I find that the vast majority of the Australian media is quick to condemn reports of healing rather than asking exploratory questions which lead to a clearer understanding. Instead, they challenge and attack as if on a witch hunt. I wonder how this helps their audience. I fail to see how anyone can discover alternative help when the information providers are biased or blind. Fortunately for me, my ability to see and read the human aura comes to my rescue most of the time.

A few years ago whilst being interviewed by John Mangos on his morning television show for the Seven Network, I called his attention to a cameraman who was in considerable pain, and suggested that he would be better served by an osteopath than the treatment currently being provided by a chiropractor. The audience were in awe when the cameraman described how a recent sporting accident had caused his problem. He welcomed my advice because his local chiropractor had relieved the pain but not cured it. John Mangos in his fairness allowed the audience to witness my ability to read auras and my desire to help, not to hinder.

During a national radio telephone interview, Stan Zemanek of 2UE asked me to describe his aura. I quickly described his current health issues. He responded by saying 'You're so accurate'. He invited me into the radio studio for a follow-up interview. During the interview he told his audience that he would be seeking a private appointment to see me.

I have crossed paths with the rich and the famous as well as the poor and the destitute. There have been some miseries and there have been exciting moments like conversing, long distance, from London to Sydney with ninety-year-old veteran actor Sir John Mills regarding his ailing wife's condition; or when treating the arthritic hands of the 1960s legendary British 'king of rock and roll', Long John Baldry, during his concert tour of Australia — a giant of a man with manners of a gentleman.

But the memory that lingers in my mind, thrilling me every time, belongs to a moment in September 1997 — a telephone call — 'Hello, may I speak to Judith Collins? It's Donovan calling'. It was the singer/composer, whose words and music first wove their way into my life when I was thirteen years old. He said that his father had suffered a stroke. I offered to fly to London if the stroke was not too debilitating because I have had success with treating the condition. But, alas his father died.

Donovan alone awakened a depth of spirituality in me. I knew that only my mother could really understand what his telephone call meant to me. So I called her. As expected she promptly recalled the times when I had protested for peace, fund-raised for the poor, worked with homeless children, counselled the desperate and cared for the elderly and the sick. She attributed these activities to Donovan's lyrics that you should 'Wear your love like heaven'.

The soundtrack which he composed for the enlightening motion picture film *Brother Sun, Sister Moon* portrayed beautifully the spiritual development and achievements of its subject, St Francis of Assisi.

People often ask me who and what have played a major role in the development of my gifts. Of course, Donovan's creativity has played a major supportive and ongoing role. William Blake, the poet and philosopher, expanded my thinking into another world. Leonardo da Vinci's forward thinking and probing thirst for an understanding of life, also inspired me.

Daily and weekly encounters continually add to my personal development. On one occasion, a middle-aged woman approached my display stall at a psychic fair in Sydney. Fascinated by the speed with which I drew and analysed the human aura she attempted to book a consultation but discovered that I was engaged for several hours. So, she sought me out during my lunch break.

I did not appreciate being invaded in this way — I needed time to relax and prepare for the onslaught of public attention during the afternoon. I therefore attempted to politely dismiss her by asking her to see me at my clinic. She stopped me in mid-sentence and recounted her story. I quickly assessed her aura for deceitfulness and found her to be truthful. Her broad English brogue set the scene for the tale.

While sitting on a railway platform in England she was approached by a man who introduced himself as Harry Edwards, medium and healer. He accurately described her family's pattern of hereditary illness and told her that when the time came for her to be healed she would be far away from England. In order to be healed she had to seek out a fair-headed woman whose name was Judith. 'You will recognise her by her clinic, which by its name reflects the care of the Earth.' After boarding the train she hurriedly wrote down all he had said. In the years following, she kept an eye out for her healer as she and her diplomat husband travelled to the far corners of the world. Now, on his retirement they had chosen to settle in Australia.

Nearing the climax of the story she asked if I was a healer. Suffering with heart disease, she had attended the show to seek natural relief as her doctors had offered little hope. When I explained that my clinic was called Earthkeepers Healing Sanctuary, her face turned ghostly white. Furthermore, little did she know that three days prior to our encounter I had been given a copy of the work of the late Harry Edwards, a famous British healer. The fickle finger of fate works in mysterious ways.

In 1997 when my secretary was planning my tour in England I requested that she secure an appointment for my injured knee to be treated by a spiritual healer named George Chapman. Many years ago he was invited by Dr Lang to become his vessel of healing. The late Dr Lang, a renowned eye surgeon in his day, wished to continue his healing service from the Spirit realm. The process is simple. George goes into a deep trance or hypnotic state of mind to allow Dr Lang to work through him.

Dr Lang invited me to lay on the healing couch and open my eyes wide so that he could ascertain the problem. He enquired, 'You have a scar on your eye. How did you do that?'. Several years ago a small piece of metal lodged in my eye. Although successfully removed by a skilful doctor, rust had caused scarring. Dr Lang held George's hands over my eyes and began moving his fingers as if performing an operation. It certainly felt like it. At the point when my eye began to sting and burn with heat, he said 'The discomfort will pass. Please close your eyes and rest them'. I felt my knee moving about internally as Dr Lang described the problem, without touching it. At that point I understood just how my clients feel when I treat them. He continued chatting, 'I see we are in the same line of work my dear. What illness do you particularly enjoy treating?'. 'Hearts, backache, infertility and arthritis,' I replied. My husband sat watching the whole episode. I walked away feeling absolutely wonderful.

The experience added a whole new dimension to my own learning because, for the first time, I had been on the receiving end.

Healing has brought a light into my life. To me there is nothing better than to witness a fellow human being or animal overcome pain and suffering.

While working in Melbourne in 1997 a stout, retired Scottish gentleman was one of the hundreds of people who needed to test me out. I liked him instantly for his honesty as he set about telling me that he didn't believe I could help him.

I retorted, 'Are you a betting man, because if you are, I'll take you on'. We broke into laughter at each other's sense of humour as he awkwardly lifted his painful knees on to the healing table. I will let him tell you the rest of the story.

> My name is Edward Mole. For many years I suffered rheumatism of the knees. I had an operation but with no lasting effect. I had given up hope of any improvement until my daughter said 'Come on, Dad. You need to see Judith Collins'. My mind asked 'What can she do that a doctor can't?' but the pain said 'Give it a go!'. So I went and saw Judith and I am glad I did. Two visits later my knees had vastly improved. By the way, she also cured my digestive problem as well.
>
> I am not a person easily swayed but I know one thing: if I have any more problems, I will go to Judith Collins.

Little did Edward know that arthritic knees normally respond quite quickly to spiritual healing. I had known I was on an 'almost certainty' when I made that bet.

Characters like Edward bring colour into my working day so I welcome them with a smile, not with a frown. Approximately one in three people seeking a personal consultation are in one form or another, sceptical or cautious. However, when pain and discomfort are dispelled, a bond between us forms.

Healing has exposed me to a wide section of the world's community. I have grown to respect the diverse range of customs and beliefs. Buddhists utter their sacred chants throughout the healing session. Some Maltese families accompany their sick loved-one to the session. Equipped with rosary beads, they pray on their knees, silently or aloud, as I heal. Most of the Italians place a picture of their favourite saint or the Virgin Mary on their chest to assist the healing. Those of the Greek and Russian orthodox churches either wear a gold cross or place a crucifix on their chest during the healing. The New Age person wears a crystal around their neck and removes all metal jewellery for fear of vibrational interference. The sceptics either confront me with their beliefs or test out my skills by way of trickery. And, on all occasions I do my best to service their needs.

The healing path which I have woven from state to state in this vast country has been paved by word of mouth. I remain fascinated as to how widespread the community of family is. When I enquired of an Adelaide woman how she came to know of me, she replied, 'Oh, I'm the nextdoor neighbour of Margaret's cousin's brother-in-law's boss's sister's godson. An intriguing network of communication indeed!

I came to heal. They come to be healed. Together we grow closer to the realisation of wholeness of our being.

2 VULNERABILITY TO ILLNESS

YOUR STATE of health is perhaps the most important thing in your entire life. Yet, the majority of people do nothing to ensure its well-being, and when their body fails to live up to their expectations, they complain. Most spend more time grooming their animals, their cars or their careers than they do contemplating whether or not their body can deliver the service required for day-to-day life. Your health is your greatest wealth. But when it goes haywire it can send you either financially, emotionally or physically bankrupt. What good is life if the body won't deliver? What is it all worth?

A client reported that three of the four medical specialists she had consulted enquired of her 'Do you drink tea, coffee, Coca Cola or alcohol? and 'Do you often eat chocolate?'. Such questions are commonly asked by the hostess of a tea party, not a doctor. The truth is that the modern person rushes to and fro to achieve their goals of a nice home, a good job and lifestyle. They tend to eat on the run or hurriedly, and have an imbalanced diet with a high sugar, salt and saturated fat content. They tend to be so busy 'doing' that they forget 'being' until tragedy occurs.

I recall a client called Bob. He was a very successful businessman who had married the girl of his dreams in his late teens. Together they produced three daughters who, in turn, produced seven grandchildren between them. Three months into retirement he felt tired and was experiencing a serious loss of appetite. He came to me and asked if I could boost his energy as he had much to do about his newly built home.

I assessed his condition and his aura and promptly advised him to see a doctor for a conclusive diagnosis. He looked me straight in the eyes and asked 'You think I have cancer, don't you?'.

He died seven months later. The cancer had practically eaten his body. Previously, he was unaware because he was too busy being busy and ignored the signals which his body had been giving him for eighteen months.

He wife was left with a brand new house with unfinished grounds, in an area far removed from relatives and friends. When he died she was isolated and alone. Six months later she sold the property at a loss so as to quickly escape her grief. The retirement, dream home and plans of travelling the world were crushed for ever.

During healing sessions he would repeatedly say to me, 'I've worked my guts out for everything I've got'. Dying from stomach and bowel cancer proved that he really did!

Over and over again I have seen the patterns of this story repeated in the lives of others and I ask myself why. What is wrong with us that we have to drive ourselves to self-destruction?

One would think that higher education and community health education programmes should have encouraged us to realise that our thinking patterns, beliefs and emotions play a vital role in maintaining health and well-being. It's unfortunate that still today, most of us do not recognise how our life experience affects the human body until chronic or terminal illness challenges and we become a witness to how the body has reacted to lifestyle and belief systems.

Anyone who has ever been frightened, worried or very nervous, knows how the stomach churns and produces a sickly feeling. Such tension may also cause frequent urination, breathlessness, restless sleep, headache, heart palpitations, flatulence or a loose bowel. This is a basic example of how thought and emotion can physically affect the body. Our vulnerability to illness is directly related to the life we lead, the food we eat, the air we breathe, the way we think and what we believe as well as the varied experiences of life and the inevitable ageing process. Some of us will suffer greatly, while others suffer very little.

More interesting is how the 'learned responses' or behaviour established in younger years present themselves as disease later on in life. Anger seems to produce ailments which infect or burn the body. Resentment deep within the mind appears to eat away at the core of the body, resulting in cancer, tumours and decay. A long term pattern of criticism restricts self-expression and produces diseases such as arthritis. Pain of varying degrees is often associated with deep-seated guilt. Patterns of revenge seem to encourage the manifestation of hereditary and contagious disease.

One of the saddest cases with which I have worked was a forty-year-old woman whose fifteen-year-old son committed suicide. Before committing the act he wrote letters to his father, brothers, grandparents and schoolmates. Two years following his death, the mother was diagnosed with ovarian cancer. Identifying patterns of guilt, I referred her to a hypnotherapist who soon revealed a self-destructive pattern. Apparently the mother took on deep-seated guilt because the son had not written to her. When I suggested the idea that perhaps he couldn't say goodbye because he loved her too much, and it hurt to say goodbye, she sobbed and sobbed endlessly. I held and rocked her gently as if nursing an infant. Her recovery from the cancer was slow but successful.

Ownership of an affliction is an obstacle. Expressions such as 'I have cancer' or 'my brain tumour' are, to me, an indication that the person has adopted the illness as an integral part of their life. When the mind recognises ownership, it's unlikely to surrender its possession without a struggle. Would you give your car or house away to anyone who asked? Would you cut off a finger because someone suggested it? No. You would have to think the request through thoroughly. It's the same principle with illness. To say, 'I feel a cold coming on' simply recognises the onset of the ailment. However, to awake each morning and search your body for symptoms is the adoption of an illness. To awake, take your medication and get on with daily life, helps you to not only combat the illness but to avoid its spread.

To alter recent and old patterns retained by the mind requires skilful persuasion. A change of diet, beliefs, thought patterns, action and new information, entice it to recognise a change in behaviour, thereby reducing or releasing the cause of disease. Here are some commonly used terms which hinder good health.

- Terminal illness — 'I am sick to death of...'
- Fatigue — 'I am sick and tired of...'
- Stomach/bowel — 'I am fed up with everything'
- Bowel/rectum/sacrum — 'It gives me the shits'
- Head/brain — 'It's a headache'
- Legs/ankles/knees — 'I just can't stand it'
- Nervous system 'It gives me the blue willies' or 'It's a pain in the neck'
- Eyes — 'I can't see for looking'
- Lungs — 'It takes my breathe away'
- Teeth — 'I'm fed up to the back teeth'
- Jaw — 'I've bitten off more than I can chew'
- Throat — 'No one listens to a thing I say' or 'Swallow your pride'
- Skeletal — 'I've bent over backwards...' or 'Sticks and stones will break my bones but names will never hurt me'
- Arthritis — 'If you play with fire, your fingers get burnt'
- Hearing — 'I've had an earful'

Monitor your beliefs by listening carefully during conversations to the words you commonly use. This will help to ascertain how your attitude is programming your physical body to respond. Further to this, examine your behaviour. Are you naturally rebellious, complacent, agreeable or weak of character? Do you harbour anger, jealousy, fear or resentment? Are you restricted by the opinions and expectations of others? In order to determine your personal pattern of debilitating stress, evaluate your sense of freedom of choice in life.

ILL AT EASE

In today's modern world the human body finds itself dumped on by the fast pace of life. Pollution (the stuff you can see and the stuff you can't see), fast food, poorer quality drinking water, excessive noise levels, a decline of social etiquette, a deterioration of social values, dysfunctional relationships, argumentative political leadership and so on — all have an influence on the disposition of the health of the physical, mental and emotional body.

NOISE

On the first day of work at my clinic in Sydney, my concentration was easily distracted by the drone of noise from buses, trucks, cars with poor exhaust systems and aeroplanes flying overhead at half-hourly intervals. The noise was so bad that at times I felt I could hardly hear myself speak. I said to a client 'I'll tell you when the aeroplane has passed us', to which he replied 'I hadn't noticed the noise overhead until you mentioned it'. While one could marvel at how the human psyche adjusts to its environment, I was left wondering whether this was a good thing or not. Curiosity caused me to test other clients that day. Disappointingly no one heard the noise except myself. Comments such as 'you'll get used to it' and 'you don't hear it after a while' alarmed me.

According to patterns displayed in the human aura, a person can tolerate consistent noise for only a brief period of time before it negatively affects both the nervous and endocrine systems. The term 'ill at ease' describes the long term effect. Where there is no ease, illness follows.

Stillness, whether achieved through surroundings, peace of mind or relaxation is an important part of self-healing. Here's how it can be achieved:
• Leave the noise behind and spend a weekend in tranquil surroundings for two to three days per month.
• Upon waking, monitor your breathing pattern. Shallow breathing can indicate stress. Follow the deep breathing exercise on page 115.
• Be alone, quiet and still, for one hour each week to promote rejuvenation.
• At least three times per week allow yourself to drift into a daydream.
• Learn to meditate. You'll be surprised how wonderful you'll feel.

- Walk along a beach or a desolate street in the early hours of a morning, before the traffic starts rolling.
- Include stillness in your daily routine. Sit perfectly still for five minutes every day.

LIFELESS FOOD

Have you noticed that food doesn't taste the way you remember it? Tomatoes lack their sweetness, and carrots, Brussels sprouts, beans, cauliflower, broccoli, broad beans and lettuce have lost their zest. Furthermore, their regular position at the dinner table is being eroded by quickly prepared, highly salted, highly sweetened so-called food stuffs.

The *Macquarie Dictionary* says that food is 'what is eaten or taken into the body for nourishment'. However, in today's world, food tends to be used more to curb the appetite than to enhance personal health and well-being. If you're feeling a bit peckish, you have a bag of potato chips or a chocolate bar. If you're thirsty you have a soft drink. And if you're hot, you have an ice cream. There's nothing very nourishing in these. A quick snack whilst out and about town was once an apple or banana.

Is it then not a sad indictment on society to be told by your doctor that you have to change your diet in order to alleviate ill health? Surely this is suggesting 'you have been poisoning and/or polluting yourself' or even worse, that 'your irresponsible behaviour has led to this disease'. Very quickly the patient learns that the local greengrocer, not the supermarket, is the place to shop. Natural health food stores are also a major asset, providing organic food and ingredients plus natural medications.

If local fruit and vegetables have lost their flavour and mostly look unappetising:
- Ask your local health food store to put you in touch with an organic fruit and vegetable supplier. Community-run networks have been operating in every state for years.
- Ask your local greengrocer to stock organically and locally grown produce.
- Contact the local council to locate community support groups which can help link you with food and aid groups

for those with conditions such as cancer, asthma, allergies and disability.

- You can even grow your own food organically as a supplement to your seasonal intake.

I began growing vegetables over twenty-five years ago. I started with a few string bean seeds and some lettuce seedlings which I planted between a few small cuttings of white geraniums. Mine was a very small garden, approximately 1 m x 0.5 m, alongside our caravan. Money was scarce. My husband was a full-time university student and at that time I was physically incapacitated with partial paralysis. I didn't even own a gardening book. I simply put the seeds in the ground, watered regularly and hoped for the best.

Because nature was good to me on my first attempt, I carried on planting a vegetable patch wherever we lived. When I learnt how to garden organically according to Esther Dean's *No Dig Garden*, crop yields increased dramatically. Then, sixteen years ago, I learnt about 'Permaculture', a natural, organic and sustainable system developed by Bill Mollison. I was hooked for life.

We sold our house, bought an old run-down, defunct, free-range chook farm, planted hundreds of trees and a home orchard, then filled it with resident caretakers (chooks, ducks and geese). We also established a large area of no-dig garden systems and a natural water system. We then sat back, enjoyed the environment and slowly reaped the benefits of our hard work and commitment. A well prepared no-dig system requires very little maintenance and can therefore easily accommodate a hectic lifestyle and physical disabilities.

It's amazing how a well planned and thoughtfully planted tiny space can produce such an abundance of food. A large pot is adequate for a tomato plant with lettuce, parsley and basil planted around it. So there is no excuse as to why we can't all improve the quality of our food intake. Supermarket-advertised 'free-range' eggs have nothing on those produced by my own chooks! For a start, mine look and taste better!

Due to public demand we open our gardens to the general public several times per year. However, visitors to the Healing Sanctuary on our property also have the opportunity to purchase free-range eggs and freshly picked seasonal fruit and vegetables, as well as breathe in nature at its best.

EMOTIONS

Discomfort of life makes human beings behave in all manner of ways. I believe that nowhere is the ever-increasing aggressiveness of society more evident than on our roads. Every day you can witness intolerance, impatience, bad manners, aggression, fear, poor concentration, lack of co-ordination, temper tantrums, power struggles and sheer carelessness. I often sit in traffic and watch these tortured souls go through their paces.

Have you ever noticed how aggressive drivers of unairconditioned cars can become in the heat of the Australian summer? They seem to want to get to their destination faster just to avoid the piping hot sun. Parking is no exception. In parking lots of large shopping malls you can see cars perched anxiously, like birds of prey, awaiting the vacating of a sheltered parking space or the opportunity to queue jump.

Frustration affects each and every one of us differently.

This brings to mind the story of a friend. While waiting in a queue at McDonald's he knew he would not be kept long because of the organisation's reputation for efficiency. However the woman standing in front of him, although only second in line from the cashier, was huffing and puffing, mumbling obscenities. She had been kept waiting less than three minutes. Her intolerance affected my friend greatly. He returned to his car and sobbed deeply for an hour because two weeks earlier he had returned from filming a documentary in Rwanda where he was forced to watch women with starving babies sit in queues for three and four days for one lousy bowl of rice. His sense of helpless despair was magnified by the woman's impatience.

Commonly, people become frustrated because of poor time management on their part, leaving things to the last minute or dawdling until there is little or no time left to achieve what they wish. This in turn raises a myriad of responses which can cause unnecessary stress.

A member of my extended family is known to be reliably late. She is invited to lunch at 12 pm if required to arrive by 1.30 pm. The family has overcome its annoyance at her inconsiderate behaviour by recognising her sheer laziness and muddle headedness and by developing a strategy to avoid stress and confrontation.

We first encounter the feeling of guilt as children as it has generally been used as a form of discipline in the rearing of children for centuries. We can therefore say that our genes have been conditioned to feeling guilty. Some people even go so far as to say that they feel guilty for being born.

Anxiety, worry, fear, resentment, anger and guilt suffocate effectiveness. I believe these emotions are also the root cause of an inability to initiate or respond to self-healing. However, overcoming them is not about undertaking a process of self-forgiveness or self-confession. It's about shifting and changing your attitude.

Throughout adolescence and early adulthood I saw my mother as a 'wet blanket', always raining on my parade. However, when I took the time to stop, observe and listen, I saw her as a fair and forthright person who offered me an honest assessment of myself. After all, she knew me well enough to do so. When I shifted my attitude — a fear of criticism — my long-term resentment was extinguished and my mother became my best friend. I also learnt that I could not define my own self-worth unless I examined the opinions of those who knew me well and why and how they had been formed. When defending our honour we often neglect to hear the real message.

What you experience in day-to-day life contributes to the development of your character. You can choose to follow the path of poor role models or you can choose to improve your lot. You can choose to see yourself as successful, or see yourself as a failure. Most people find it is easier to whinge, whine and complain rather than to make necessary changes. My father, a hard-working man and devoted husband, was of the old school. His wife didn't work. She reared the children, kept house and was there for him. Fortunately he married a woman whose goal was to do just that.

While in my teens, I realised that this pattern was not for me. I was emerging as a woman of the sixties — equal pay, equal rights, equal power. However, the pattern I chose to keep was my parents' ideal — ensuring that you marry your best friend so you can both enjoy each other's company and share in everything you do.

What family patterns have you kept and discarded?

THE STRESS CONTRIBUTION

In the modern world it is almost impossible to escape stress factors. Through my experience as a healer I have reached the conclusion that stress in its many guises plays an active role in the cause of disease. While I believe there is positive stress, the kind that motivates and provokes affirmative action, negative stress is more recognisable because of its restrictive and debilitating effect on the psychological and physical body. Obvious symptoms of stress are as follows:

- Sleeplessness
- Shortness of breath
- A racing heart
- Frequent changes in body temperature
- Vulnerability to criticism
- Emotional outbursts
- Quick temper or violent temper
- Poor concentration span
- Frequent colds and coughs
- Stomach and bowel distress

When left untreated for a number of years any one of these symptoms can accelerate or trigger illness.

As a youngster Mary noticed that she became constipated when stressed during exam time or when she was required to socialise with strangers. Although the constipation reduced in its severity as social skills were mastered, her bowels became tied up in knots whenever she was challenged. On reaching thirty-four years of age she was diagnosed as having irritable bowel syndrome. Fortunately she responded to spiritual healing and was cured within three treatments.

DIET OF PEACEFULNESS

Rest is universally recognised as being vitally important to good health yet most people flout it. The average person works all year, hungering for a block of weeks in which to laze at home, undertake renovations, re-arrange the garden, float in the pool in the backyard or catch up with things that have escaped them all year. Then, whenever finances allow, a holiday trip is planned. All in all, however, the hustle and bustle continues to some extent.

Creating peacefulness is not about resting your head on a pillow for half an hour; nor is it sitting comfortably reading the newspaper. It's about creating a haven in your garden or in your house where you can contemplate and meditate. Peacefulness is about stillness — the deep inner silence that only day-dreaming and meditation can offer to the mind, body and spirit. Peacefulness is where the mind is no longer twisted with worry or taunted by ambition and ego, but stands quiet and still; where the nervous system comes to rest and where you come to see the unique value of being you.

I'm filled with dismay when I hear people say: 'I can't meditate. My mind won't be still. It won't shut up'. Or even worse, they say 'I can't concentrate or get the right focus'. How sad! Such words speak for themselves but indicate stress and being ill at ease.

A diet of peacefulness is essential for our well-being and for a feeling of wholeness. It helps us to maintain a balance in life.

Here, it is fitting to quote the words of the great Australian poet Dame Mary Gilmore:

> These are the little shoes that died.
> We could not keep her still.
> But all day long her busy feet
> danced to her eager will.
>
> Leaving the body's loving warmth
> the spirit ran outside;
> then from the shoes they slipped her feet,
> And the little shoes died.

When I was a little girl my grandmother taught me to live each day as if it were my last — somehow and somewhere to find the beauty and love in life. This caring and gentle being indirectly taught me that every moment that passes us by is lost forever and can never be replaced. Time lost is not misplaced but wasted. Life is a matter of time. Some live it well and long; others short but sweet. Unfortunately, many mask it with activity and then wonder where it has gone.

My dying patients have taught me the meaning of time: the string of moments that capture the meaning of a life when the life itself has gone. How important it is to be at peace with yourself before passing over. I therefore advocate that peacefulness is the most vital ingredient in your daily regime.

BOREDOM AND INEFFECTIVENESS

My son wanted to complete the last two years of his schooling at boarding school. So, I had him investigate all the schools which appealed to him and choose one. The principal of the chosen school suggested to my son that perhaps he was seeking a boarding position because he was the only child living at home and was bored. As my son responded with a grin I suggested an explanation was owed to the principal. He quoted our family motto: 'Boredom is when the mind is too lazy to guide or entertain the body'. I explained that we don't have boredom in our home. Instead we replace it with the insight to either change an activity, the scenery or the company we keep.

* Boredom is an unconstructive use of time.
* It is the procrastinator of life.
* It erodes inspiration and creative impulses.

At the age of nine my son learnt this lesson for himself. It had rained solidly for a fortnight. He sat staring out of the glass French doors of our back verandah, wondering what next to do with himself. When I enquired what was the matter he suggested that he was bored. With that I grabbed hold of his hand tightly, flung open the doors and jumped off the verandah and into the torrential rain, taking him with me. With gaiety, I dragged him, skipping up and down our long driveway, stopping to jump in all the puddles which the downpour had created. Within a few minutes he had captured the spirit of the moment and began laughing and splashing me. We shook the bushes and the trees to create waterfalls. Arm in arm, skipping and hopping along we sang: 'Here we are again, happy as can be. All good friends, in jolly good company'. No longer was he bored. Instead he had created a lasting memory.

My husband met us at the back door with large beach towels, a hot drink and grilled cheese on toast — a fitting conclusion to a spontaneous moment in life which created an everlasting memory. Nowadays, the moment anyone mentions the word 'boredom' we look at each other and laugh.

RELATING TO ONE ANOTHER

While it is true that we live in a time of prosperity, there exists a poverty of love and respect. Simple courtesies of yesteryear seem to have disappeared. Rarely do you see a young person give an old lady their seat on a bus or someone help an elderly person to cross the road.

I remember standing in a queue waiting for service in a large department store. A mentally disabled young man was attempting to buy his mother a birthday present. The necklace cost $3.80 and he was twenty cents short. In the most polite tone he asked if he could return the owed money when he got his pension next week. After being abruptly dismissed and escorted to the floor supervisor, he repeated his request in a gentle voice. Glaring at him as if he was the carrier of some contagious disease, she stepped back and growled: 'The price is the marked price and that's it! I'm busy. Don't bother me'. At that point I cut in and gave him the twenty cents. If looks could kill, the floor supervisor would be guilty of my murder. Her aura revealed a very angry person. She had made the wrong choice of husbands and for the past twenty years had felt sentenced for life. I could see arthritic patterns manifesting due to her long term anger.

In another instance, a very sickly woman, riddled with cancer and unresponsive to chemotherapy, was brought to me by her adult daughters as a last resort. One daughter told the tale of how her mother was still expected by her father to clean the house, cook, wash the dishes and do the shopping. No member of the family had visited her at home for six years because of his hostile nature. As the woman was too weak to travel, I sent one of my healing assistants to treat her at home. However, that system of treatment soon came to an end when the father, returning from work early, erupted and physically dragged my assistant out of their home.

This caused me to promptly telephone each of the daughters and ask: 'How much do you love your mother? If you leave her there she'll surely die'. I had noticed in the mother's aura that her only relief from the trauma of life was to die. She had begun to die as a young wife and mother. It was just a matter of time before the body would allow her wishes to be fulfilled.

The daughters packed up her belongings while their husbands stood guard. Despite the dysfunction in the family the bond she had established with her children was able to save her life. Today the woman has regained her self-identity, is completely healed of cancer, has a part-time job (her first ever) and takes great pleasure in the rearing of her grandchildren.

Because all of us need to be needed and want to be liked and appreciated, we easily fall prey to emotional despair. Sooner or later we have to develop skills to defend ourselves from the trauma. Some of us learn to scream and shout, while others crawl into their shell. Some learn to please, while others outwardly rebel or inwardly resent being told what to do. It is a skill to learn how to respond to rejection, criticism, jealousy and resentment in a positive way so as not to be affected.

THE TOXIC COCKTAIL

Whether you are taking vitamin tablets, herbs or prescribed drugs you need to be fully aware of their long term benefits and any possible side effects. For example, my mother, who was experiencing tightness of the chest and a sudden loss of energy, discovered that the high blood pressure tablets which she had taken every day for the past nine years had quite devastating side effects such as hardening of the arteries.

Frequently I am having to heal people suffering from the side effects of some prescribed drugs. Just as you decide what to eat daily, it is the responsibility of the patient to say yes or no to medication and to fully understand its effects on the human body.

A client suffering with multiple sclerosis told me how her doctor wanted to prescribe a drug whose side effects, when researched, read worse than the disease itself. Of course, she declined to take the drug. A nursing sister by profession she was accustomed to analysing medications.

In another case, one unfortunate fellow was prescribed three cortisone tablets per day instead of three per week. The side effects were horrendous. His body blew up like a balloon, his breathing was restricted and major organs were badly affected.

A doctor friend said to me, 'Just remember, no one is infallible'. So, safeguard yourself. Know what you are subjecting your body to so that you are aware of the 'desired' outcome.

HEREDITARY PATTERNS

So, Great Grandma was the problem was she? There always seems to be someone to blame for long-standing family weaknesses and illness. My beloved grandfather died of stomach cancer when I was a young child. My grandmother died of a cerebral haemorrhage. They were both under sixty years old. Another grandfather died of wear and tear. He was in his late eighties. My remaining grandmother is a lively chatterbox in her mid-nineties. My own father has had a double by-pass surgery and cancer cut. My mother has high blood pressure, has had a hysterectomy and suffered a mild stroke. This gives me a clear picture of what to correct in my life if I am to avoid the severity of hereditary weakness.

Eighteen years ago I made a conscious decision to change my family patterns through diet and lifestyle. Whilst it's true I lead a more hectic lifestyle, I choose to live in a less polluted and crowded environment. I meditate regularly and practise deep breathing. I grow and eat organic foods. I drink filtered water. I sing all the time and laugh constantly. Despite this, I have the same round shape of my forebears. I comfort myself by knowing I am positively contributing to a change in hereditary patterns.

My husband, who is slowly losing his hair, is proud that our lifestyle has allowed him to keep his hair some twenty years longer than his father and fifteen years longer than his younger brother. He says 'It's one thing to be bald when you are a young man and another when you are middle aged'.

THE FAMILY HEALTH TREE

To determine your hereditary traits and vulnerability to illness, complete the Family Health Tree. The diagram should present a clear and concise picture, to see which patterns you need to change and correct, so as to avoid personal illness, and its spread to future generations.

WHAT TO RECORD
• Name of family member; • Age at death; • Cause of death; • Illness experienced during lifetime; • Surgical operations.

Family Health Tree

Grandmother	Grandfather	Grandmother	Grandfather
Arthritis Asthma Poor eyesight Headaches	Bad back Weak bladder Varicose veins Bowel cancer Died aged 79	Diabetes Dementia High blood pressure Stroke Difficult births Died aged 69	Arthritis, Sinus Susceptible to colds Gout Died in sleep aged 81

Mother	Father
Sinus, Asthma Irritable bowel Poor eyesight	Heart bypass Arthritis Died aged 61

YOU
Diabetes
High blood pressure
Failing eyesight

ASTROLOGICAL HEALTH PATTERNS

I have come to recognise the truth of astrological health patterns. Each astrological star sign has its own unique strengths and weaknesses which affect different parts of the physical body.

Aries: head, face, upper jaw, cerebrum and cerebrospinal system.
Taurus: ears, vocal chords, neck and throat, palate, salivary glands, cerebellum.
Gemini: hands, arms, shoulders, nervous system, upper respiratory system.
Cancer: breasts, diaphragm, stomach and skin.
Leo: heart, back and spine.
Virgo: abdomen, small and large intestines, pancreas, spleen, metabolic system.
Libra: kidneys, lumbar spine, ovaries, descending colon.
Scorpio: nose, genitals, blood, urethra, bladder.
Sagittarius: hips, thighs, liver, veins, the muscular system.
Capricorn: teeth, skeletal system, knees.
Aquarius: lower legs and ankles, circulatory system.
Pisces: feet, toes, lymphatic system.

Dawn's story — Debilitating knee pain

As an astrologer, it has long been clear to me that using my knowledge of astrology to determine a method of healing is beneficial to the health of me and my family. One such example of combining astrology with the benefits of spiritual healing concerns the problems I encountered with my knee.

The pain in my knee was at times unbearable. Many a night my sleep was disturbed due to the constant pain and swelling, the cause of which I was at a loss to find. To walk long distances was a challenge, resulting in severe pain and discomfort. The use of my knee would make it swell considerably, taking two or three days of rest to bring the swelling down. As long as I didn't use my knee and led a very passive life, I found I could cope for short periods of time. Then the situation would return when I became more active.

My experience as an astrologer compelled me to look at my personal chart in an endeavour to seek the catalyst and, as a result, find a solution to my problem. Astrologically, being an Aries, knees should not be a problem as Aries rules the head. However, this was not the case in my situation.

When analysing my chart, several aspects (relationships between the planets) allowed me to see the situation more clearly. The transiting planet Pluto, the major transformer of self and situations, was making a heavy aspect to the planets Saturn and Uranus (Saturn representing bones and limitations (among other things) and Uranus representing freedom and movement). Thus, the position of Pluto was stressing my ability to move around, forcing me to make change.

Paradoxically, Pluto is also the 'Great Healer'. It is the ruler of the eighth house (spiritual healing, birth, death and psychology). With these insights I was able to conclude that the solution to my problem was spiritual healing. Having heard of Judith Collins' healing powers I made an appointment to see her for a healing session.

During the appointment at Judith's 'Earthkeepers' I lay on the table and Judith worked on my knee, all the time just chatting to me about everyday occurrences. However, the sensation I felt in and around my knee was a deep penetrating heat. The feeling of this heat can only be described as being wrapped in a beautiful, warm, soft bubble. When Judith stopped working on my knee the feeling lasted for several hours. Simultaneously there was a feeling of a cool breeze around the knee.

The healing relieved the pain, enabling me to be reasonably active. A few weeks later I decided to visit Judith again for healing as the knee was still on the tender side, though much improved. Since the second visit to Judith I can honestly say I have had no more swelling or sleepless nights.

Out of interest, on my original visit to Judith she told me that my knee problem was due to an old injury that occurred years ago. At the time I could not remember any related incident. A few days later I remembered that twenty-five years prior I had tripped over a hose at the bottom of the back steps and hit my knee, causing pain and swelling for a few days.

Often we feel perplexed by the nature and source of our health issues. Astrology allows us to see our vulnerabilities by indicating the triggers, time, nature and often the source of our problems. In this way a familiarity with our Natal Charts can give us comfort in the knowledge of what we can expect to confront in our lives. Personally, it gives me peace of mind to know that these occurrences are part of my life plan.

THE INNER ENERGY (CHAKRAS)

The spinning, coloured, cone-shaped energy centres known as chakras are an integral part of the auric body. They absorb and distribute its vibrant energy to different parts of your physical body and are partially responsible for its maintenance. It could be said that they supply the body with its life-force. When one or more chakras malfunctions or becomes blocked, depression and or disease usually follow.

There are seven major chakras. Each is approximately seven to eight centimetres in diameter. Numerous minor chakras are scattered about the physical body and are approximately two to three centimetres in diameter. They each have a specific colour and role to play in relation to the body's organs and their well-being. I have highlighted the fourteen chakras, major and minor, in the illustration on page 35.

The **Earth chakra** is located approximately twenty centimetres under the feet. Consequently, as you walk barefoot on the grass the chakra becomes embedded in the earth, giving off a sense of connectedness. It governs bonding and a sense of community.

The **Feet chakra** regulates the flow of the body's energies. It governs balance, wholeness and the logical part of the mind.

The **Knee chakra** (minor) is centred at the back of each knee and monitors the flow of the body's energies. Each governs strength of purpose plus shoulder and neck muscles.I

The **Hand chakra** (minor) is centred in the palm of each hand. These chakras govern creative learning and expression.

The **Root chakra** (major) is seated at the base of the spine. It represents the 'earth' element and gives a sense of being planted firmly on the ground. It governs the adrenals, kidneys, spinal column and solid matter of the body: teeth, nails and bones. The sense of smell is also associated with the root chakra.

The **Sacral chakra** (major) is directly aligned with the sacrum on the spine and gives a sense of smooth flow of self. It relates to the water of the body: urine, vaginal fluids, semen and saliva. I have noticed in my healing practice that clients who are blocked at this level have varying degrees of arthritis or pain due to friction. The sacral chakra also governs the reproductive system.

The **Solar Plexus chakra** (major) is located on the spine at the level of the stomach. Here we experience warmth, joviality and the quality of expansion and contraction. Its fiery element relates to the brightness of what we perceive. One moment we can see our life as full and satisfying, but the next moment we see it as mundane and unsuccessful. This is an example of how the solar plexus chakra, when fluctuating, affects you.

It governs the absorption of food. When a client complains to me of sluggishness, the solar plexus is blocking their ability to absorb the nourishment of their food intake. Hence, there is no fire to kindle the flame of life! The solar plexus governs the pancreas, liver, gall bladder, stomach and nervous system.

The **Heart chakra** (major) is located on the spine at the level of the breastbone. It represents the air element. At this level you experience airiness, mobility, lightness, gentleness and social interaction. Therefore relationships have a major impact on this chakra. In my work with AIDS sufferers I have noticed that the heart chakra is usually blocked. The heart chakra governs the circulatory system, vagus nerve, heart and blood.

The **Throat chakra** is positioned on the spine at the level of the throat. Here we experience the sense of solitude. It is a vital link between expression and thought. It represents the ability to communicate with the world around us. It can be gentle and caring. When there is a poor flow of energy in this region you may be over-critical of others and disrespectful of others' opinions. Most throat conditions that I have healed fall into two categories: those who don't speak up for themselves and those who have too much to say. The two extremes seem to affect one's health. The throat chakra governs the thyroid, bronchial and vocal apparatus, the lungs and alimentary canal.

The **Third Eye chakra** is also known as the Brow Centre due to its position at the point on the forehead approximately between the eyebrows. This is the level at which the intuitive, imaginative and spontaneous self is linked to the mortal self of mind. It represents the power to materialise thought. For example, you are unhappy at work. You feel you need a change. Next morning you see the perfect job advertised in the newspaper. You arrange an interview during which you are offered the job on the spot.

The third eye governs the pituitary gland, left eye, lower brain, ears, nose and nervous system. I have noticed that in childless couples, one or both partners have stifled the imaginative self due to restrictions of one sort or another. This causes a block in the third eye. When successfully treated, a child may be conceived.

In the intuitively aware person, this chakra is expanded with rays of indigo penetrating several layers of the aura.

The **Crown chakra** is situated at the top of the head in alignment with the pineal gland. It is the mystical, spiritual link to God. When a person is enlightened, the crown chakra radiates a violet-pearl glow around the head area, commonly recognised as a halo. When a person is in excellent health the energy of the crown chakra irradiates waves of light.

The **Divine chakra** is located above the soul chakra but the distance above it varies between individuals. Its function is to maintain a permanent link to creation and to the creator. When we die, this chakra expands fully to ensure our return to the Spirit realm.

During the process of meditation the chakras open and

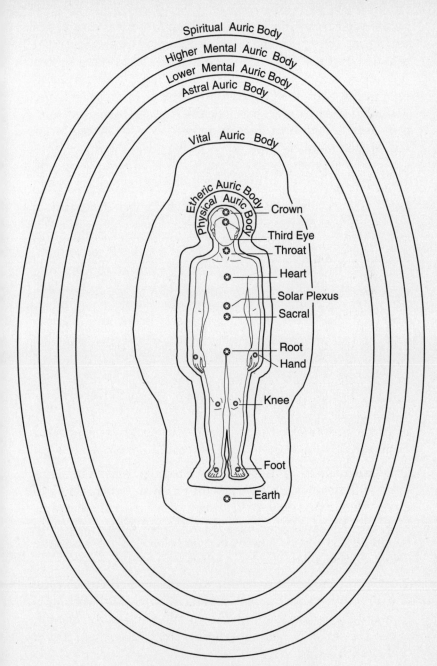

Chakras and the Human Aura

contract, displaying a beautiful array of colour that looks something like a peacock's tail feathers when fanned. Energy is like water; it follows the path of least resistance. As the muscles relax and the thinking process quietens, the physical layer of the aura spills over into the etheric layer, giving rise to a sense of self-expansion. The body senses begin to tingle and warm as your consciousness connects to the etheric layer and expands into all other levels of the aura. When the consciousness connects with the higher mental layer which in turn stimulates the spiritual auric bodies, inspiration as well as Divine guidance flows freely.

The only time that this process occurs differently is when a person is suffering from a physical or emotional illness or both. The consciousness, on reaching a state of relaxation, locks into the physical layer of the aura and draws healing from it to the physical body. An individual will usually feel this energy exchange as a sudden, sharp pain that passes rapidly. It also causes tight muscles to twitch as they release their hold on the skeletal body. A warm flow of energy can be felt around the diseased areas of the body.

Meditation not only relaxes the body and frees it from degenerative stress but it also creates a peaceful state of mind. This in turn allows a balancing of mind and body and development of the soul to take place.

3

THE GIFT OF HEALING

CLIENT AND HEALER WORKING TOGETHER

I BELIEVE THAT healing begins with the commitment of the client and the genuine interest of the health practitioner. Together, they unite resources to bring about the best possible result. Whether the practitioner be a qualified doctor or a qualified naturopath or masseur, clear attention to detail is vital.

The media tell us that more and more people are turning to natural health. I believe this is true but not just for the reasons they state. I believe people are looking for quality time and quality attention. Medication is one thing. Time to care and share is another. It's a pity that often huge financial overheads or public demand due to popularity, have turned most general practitioner surgeries into something like an assembly line. Long waiting periods followed by a five to ten minute consultation are more common than not.

I remember an occasion when I apologised to an elderly arthritic client for keeping her waiting for twenty minutes. She replied 'It's alright. Yesterday I waited two hours to see my doctor. Usually, you never keep me waiting'. That's because I value time and respect people. When you are sick and in pain, the last thing you feel like doing is sitting in a waiting room for hours. The late Mr John Livingstone once said to me 'I've spent more time waiting than being treated. Perhaps that's why I'm dying'. Who could argue with those words? I believe that constant, long waiting periods shows a lack of respect for the patients.

The stress of transport and waiting around does nothing to enhance one's ability to respond to healing. The psyche is frustrated or depressed and therefore less responsive.

When my clients are running late for their appointment, I have them sit still for five to ten minutes to regain their composure. Or, if they are very, very late, I take them through a series of deep breathing exercises to relieve their anxiety and embarrassment. The last thing one needs is to be riddled with pent-up emotion. I then direct the healing through the skull to reduce the resistance caused by anxiety.

HOW SPIRITUAL HEALING WORKS

As the healing flows forth from its Divine source it gently filters through the healer's crown chakra, then down through the pineal gland of the third eye chakra and into the hand chakras. The electromagnetic particles which make up the human aura cause the sensation of a warm, faint electrical current. I am fully aware of when I am near a person who is not well because my hands suddenly feel warm and begin to tingle.

When healing is summoned by either the healer or the client, their intuitive faculties known as the spirit mind, work in harmony with the physical mind. Using the brain as a conductor, Divine healing is directed through the body's network of intelligences — from thoughts and emotions to our very cells — to treat the cause of an ailment and to alter its programmed responses. Spiritual healing therefore calms, and alters attitudes and behavioural responses as it treats the cause of an ailment.

EXPOSING MYTHS ABOUT RECEPTIVITY TO HEALING

A belief in spiritual healing is not necessary. I have proven this time and time again with countless clients of all ages in my healing practice.

```
                    1
                 Physical
         Healing of the physical body

                    2
                Emotional
          Healing of the emotions
                    3
                 Mental
            Change or expansion
           of attitude and beliefs

                    4
                Intuitive
             Living intuitively
          and not by strict routine

                    5
                  Spirit
                 Taking on
        a new dimension of beliefs
```

The Five Levels of Balance to bring about a cure

Religious commitment is not necessary. Healing does not discriminate. It heals those who are meant to be healed whether you are a believer or not!

Being stress free and relaxed prior to healing is not necessary. Healing alleviates and/or removes the stress from the nervous system as well as the area being healed.

Meditative skills are not required. Healing flows directly to the cause of the ailment and does not require your focus. However it helps to be attuned to your body.

Jewellery does not have to be removed prior to a healing session. The belief that it interferes with the healing flow is totally incorrect. I have never asked anyone to remove their jewellery yet have brought about healing in countless people.

PREPARATION FOR HEALING

To prepare for spiritual healing one need only be content

and happy to meet with your healer. Contentment helps to stabilise the nervous system and reduce pressure within the adrenal glands, allowing you to relax and have an open mind to the healing.

Whether lying on my healing couch or sitting upright in a chair, my clients are asked to close their eyes, take several deep breaths to relax the chest and stomach muscles, and attune to their senses so that they can report all bodily sensations experienced during the healing.

FEELING THE HEALING ENERGY

The energy which is channelled through my hands, fine tunes its flow and temperature to suit the condition and ailment of the client. Therefore the sensations experienced during healing vary with the ratio of disease and pain and in accordance with the disposition of the client. One patient diagnosed with breast cancer, Aleta Garlick, said: 'During the first session with Judith I experienced incredible heat in the face and neck areas. I experienced many sensations such as tingling, pressure over the ailment and a feeling like arrows shooting through the breast'.

Hot energy is a powerful source which unblocks congestion, reduces the toxicity of organs and treats internal bruising and inflammation, blood disorders, cancerous cells and tumours. During a healing session the heat can build up in three to four minutes to become a little uncomfortable. At this point, I usually jest and tell my clients to grind their teeth until it passes.

Warm energy is a steady healing flow which motivates the body to generate self-healing via the lymph glands and immune system as well as stimulate the senses. It makes the healing process an enjoyable experience. Something like an afternoon nap. This type of energy is commonly experienced in the treatment of most ailments.

Cool energy slows the patterns of thoughts and emotions and is deeply relaxing. It is very beneficial in cases of contagious and spreading diseases. The nervous system also responds well to cool energy.

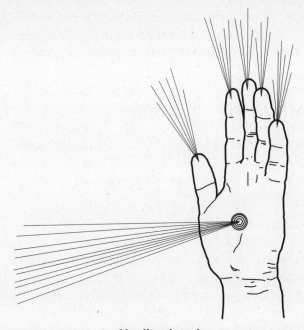

Healing hands

- Hands are the instrument of healing, nurturing and caring both for ourselves and each other.
- When activated by a healing force, the chakra centres in the palm of the hand sprays very fine beams of light from both the centre and the tips of the fingers.
- Hands move in soothing and caring ways.

Cold energy causes a condition to stabilise. Some clients say that it's like having ice cubes placed inside of you. The energy tends to hold a condition long enough in one spot for it to be targeted by the healing.

A twenty-three year old university student was brought to me by his mother. A brain tumour threatened his life. The healing energy was icy cold, causing both him and me to shiver. The active tumour in his head ceased throbbing after five more healing sessions. His next CAT scan showed decaying cells around the tumour. This told me that the cold energy had frozen its life-force. Three months later a subsequent CAT scan showed the tumour had completely shrivelled up and died.

Heavy energy places you in a trance-like state not unlike an anaesthetic. The body feels so heavy that you cannot move. A client exclaimed 'I felt like a two tonne dead weight'. This form of energy is common in long-standing illness.

Light energy alters the reality of the client. It mostly occurs when a person is ready to release their illness and also in the treatment of psychological disorders. An even lighter energy is Divinely projected when a person is approaching death. A number of clients with terminal illness call on my services for pain relief and for courage to let go and die. When light energy healing is given to grieving relatives it relieves their emotional suffering.

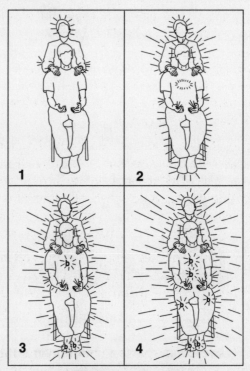

Healing progression

1 Two minutes – The healing begins to flow as the healer and client attune to the healing.
2 Five minutes – The healing communicates with the intelligences of the body.
3 Ten minutes – The healing is addressing core issues.
4 Fifteen minutes – The healing has saturated the body.

SENSATIONS AFTER HEALING

Following a healing session, spiritual healing stays in your body for four to five days and continues to work. Little sensation is felt but occasionally dramatic effects can cause one or more of the sensations which I have listed below.

An example of such an effect is given here. Frustrated by her condition, Evelyn Hartmann sought my help. She says:

> I'm a forty-year-old registered nurse, diagnosed with heart palpitations and irritable bowel syndrome. When Judith laid her hands on my head I could feel a burning in my eyes and a tightness in my forehead. When I came home that day I was extremely tired and felt a quick stabbing pain in my head. That night I had awfully painful stomach cramps which prompted several visits to the toilet.

This proved to be the first stage of Evelyn's successful healing process. On her last visit to me, the heart palpitations had completely ceased to exist and the bowel condition was well on the way to being rectified.

Tiredness experienced directly after the healing indicates that the body is slowing down so that it can fully absorb the healing and allow it to work at a steady rate throughout the entire body, activating its ability to self-heal. My clients frequently report sleeping deeply for several hours following a healing session, then awakening to find pain relief or a complete cure.

Sudden Hot Flush indicates either the expulsion of unwanted toxins, pain, locked muscles, a congested organ or a re-balancing of hormones. Prostate disorders, when treated by a spiritual healer often cause a series of hot flushes for anything up to three days.

Excessive Body Heat displays a continuation of the healing process often associated with the liver, pancreas, kidneys, adrenal and endocrine systems.

One client, Shawna McCoy, awoke the morning after her healing session for thyroid cancer and found that the skin around her throat was bright red and hot to touch. Subsequent healing sessions produced the same result. It wasn't long before it was discovered that the cancer had healed, much to the surprise of her and her doctors.

Pain is often a sign of the shift or release of deep-rooted ailments. A long term ailment can produce unbearable pain before it completely disappears. Subsequent healing sessions bring balance and pain relief.

Tingling indicates a shift in blood flow or cellular regeneration. It produces a tickling sensation within the body. Clients with leukemia often experience a sensation of pins and needles throughout the body during a healing session.

Dragging/drawing is often the feeling associated with an ailment slowly clearing or when an organ is stretching or unblocking. The sensation is commonly experienced when either the liver, kidneys, stomach or intestinal areas have been treated. This uncomfortable feeling can last for up to sixteen days as the ailment heals.

Gurgling indicates a cleansing of the spleen, stomach and /or the intestines.

Lightness is a wonderful state of consciousness indicating an emotional and physical shift. Clients are often heard saying something like 'I have a sense that there is more to life than the way I am living'. This experience commonly leads to spiritual growth.

Inner calm is a stabilising of the emotional cause of disease. I have come to recognise this as the foundation of a holistic healing process. Many of my clients report a change in disposition. To me, inner calm helps to facilitate change within oneself.

CREATING A HEALING ENVIRONMENT

CHARGING THE ATMOSPHERE

Because I feel that a hospitable and inviting atmosphere psychologically assists both the healer and the client, I put a great deal of effort into creating a restful environment to encourage both my clients and myself to be at ease. A healing environment is filled with colour, the echo of inspiring music and the subtle scents of the world around.

To further charge the atmosphere I set aside a specific room in which I work, so as to maintain a balanced, healing vibration. When healing is repeatedly conducted in an area it flows more readily and smoothly.

FENG SHUI

It makes perfect sense to ensure harmony and balance when working with vibrational energy every day. Our earliest ancestors ensured their survival by interpreting the messages of the Earth. When, later in history, they settled to farm and raise stock, these skills remained just as vital.

I personally believe that a number of disorders which stem from the nervous system are caused or worsened by exposure to an imbalance of electro-magnetic fields caused by the closeness of electrical appliances in areas where householders spend a large part of their resting time. In his book *Feng Shui — The Key Concepts*, George Birdsall explains how imbalance occurs and provides simple steps to avoid imbalance in both your living and working environments.

In my practice I have come to realise that when the healing energy flows with the Earth's natural vibration, it increases its potency. Consequently I always bring to balance the environment within my consultations rooms.

COLOUR

Colours in my consultation rooms have been specifically chosen for their ability to facilitate healing. I feel that the harshness of clinical white walls call out to be coloured in with colourful ornaments or other elements. Not only do soft soothing colours create a similar tone in the atmosphere but they have been proven to communicate with our psyche. You can determine the type of atmosphere you wish to create by referring to the effects of the following colours.

- **Apricot** and **cream** in combination create a gentle, feminine environment.
- **Pastel** and **apple-green** calm and soothe tension.
- **Pale blue** and **lavender blue** in combination stimulate our intuitiveness, helping us to be more internally sensitive.

- **Lemon-yellow** stimulates thinking and discernment.
- **Pink** and **blue** in combination enhance the child within and may stimulate memory recall.
- **Cream, amber** and **brownish tones** will help to rectify psychological disorders.

MUSIC

Music alone can set the mood of the moment, and the mood of the people. Throughout history, it has been used to heal, to protest, to boost one's confidence, to inspire faith, to incite a riot and to spread and enhance propaganda during wartime. Because music is flexible it is easily enlisted by a cause.

To me, music takes the hard edge off silence, by colouring it with pulses and harmonies. A string of musical notes may cause you to reach deep into reflection, then herald forth into unexpected delights of elation.

If you refer to 'Recommended Listening' on page 127, you will find a list of music which I have tried, tested and proved to be ideal for a healing environment.

AROMATHERAPY

Aromatherapy oils help to enhance a healing environment by gently perfuming the air to address specific needs. Avoid polluting the room's atmosphere with smoke by using an electric burner rather than one lit by candle.

Here is a list of appropriate aromatherapy oils to be burned whilst healing.

Relaxing tension in a patient: *Frankincense* slows breathing and induces a meditative state. *Sandalwood* is very calming and moderately grounding.

Balancing as a necessary part of healing: *Vetiver* has a balancing action. It is very good for bringing the body's energy into alignment and also for harmonising the energies of both the healer and patient.

Creativity and self-love: *Rose* is used for the patient who requires new direction and self-understanding.

Spirituality: *Rosemary* is used to clear rooms of imbalanced energies. It also promotes mental clarity. However, it is not suitable to be used around pregnant women. *Juniper* is a physical detoxifier.

SPONTANEOUS HEALING

Often we hear the term 'spontaneous remission' used by doctors when a disease displays signs of receding naturally. However, they frequently expect the problem to return within a two to three year period. It is at this point that conventional medicine and spiritual healing beg to differ.

When my clients announce a 'spontaneous cure' they never expect it to return. They report that their health has been amended, as well as their disposition and attitude to life. In short, a major change has come about.

I have had an ongoing fascination with the process of spontaneous healing primarily because I would like to help produce such results for every client I treat. Whilst I am aware the healing power is not mine to give each day, I work towards greater insight.

There is nothing more heart-rending than to watch a young mother trying to come to terms with who will care for and raise her children when she is dead and gone. The same can be said about a young dying person who has hardly begun to live. Each day my life is challenged by an inner desire to help all who seek me out.

In search of a satisfactory answer, I have closely monitored my clients' response to healing by assessing their medical history, self-esteem, ability to relax, attitude to life in general, religious beliefs, job satisfaction, relationship skills, childhood trauma, financial status, education and ability to handle change.

However, after all these years the process still baffles me a little. Take, for instance, two people suffering migraine, which may stem from exactly the same cause and last for the same time. One person may be totally cured in one healing session while the other may take up to twenty healing sessions to see a shift in the intensity of the headaches or to be cured outright.

Whilst there does not appear to be any specific factor that

determines whether a client will respond to spontaneous healing, there are, however, some common characteristics of clients who produce positive outcomes or who gain further insight into themselves. You need:

1 the strength to handle change in your life.
2 a secure emotional foundation in your family.
3 others to believe in you.
4 the encouragement and the support of those who care about you.
5 a fair self-esteem.
6 to feel secure in at least one section of your life.
7 to believe in tomorrow.

Brad, a man in his late thirties, came to me complaining of a long-standing pattern of headaches and back pain. His stress levels were high for several reasons: a recently failed marriage, the stress of running his own business and shallow breathing due to a smoking addiction. While awaiting a divorce and property settlement, Brad lived with his mother who encouraged him to consult me. I'll let Brad complete the story.

> I was fortunate enough to be encouraged to see Judith Collins for treatment on my back in October 1997.
>
> The nature of my ailment was a very bad back, due to an injury through playing soccer some seventeen years ago. As a result of the injury, headaches and pain were an everyday occurrence. Many years of excessive physiotherapy and chiropractic treatment were to no avail.
>
> I only had one treatment for my back. Since that day I have, without a doubt, lived pain-free.

In Brad we see enough personal stress to emotionally block his receptivity to healing. Nevertheless, Brad was healed spontaneously. Safe in the realm of his roots (mother) he was psychologically secure enough to be receptive. Furthermore, the ups and downs of private enterprise had taught him to roll with the punches and to have faith that 'tomorrow' will deliver the goods. At his deepest core he believed in his ability to create his own destiny, no matter what the odds were.

Another interesting pattern of spontaneous healing that prompts me to believe in the points which I have already outlined, is how a propensity to be spontaneously healed appears to run in close-knit families. The McLean family of Bowral in New South Wales is one such family whose story is told by Margaret, the grandmother.

Margaret's story — Weight loss and abdominal pain

In May 1994 my health started to deteriorate and my weight loss was dramatic. Having previously had ovarian cancer in 1962 and breast cancer in 1989, I naturally thought the cancer had returned.

After seeing four different doctors and having numerous tests (X-rays, CAT scans, colonoscopies), they decided to operate and investigate the cause of the weight loss and the dull ache I had in my abdomen.

After the surgery I continued to lose weight and became so weak I could not sit up at the table to eat. The doctors continued to treat me with antibiotics and anti-bacterial tablets until such time as I developed a gastric ulcer, making me even more uncomfortable.

Everyone, including myself, was quite convinced that I did not have long to live. My nephew rang me and said 'Aunty Marg, you are going to die if you don't get down to Earthkeepers Healing Sanctuary at Thirlmere and see the naturopath'.

My husband Jack took me down to see Jayne Elder the naturopath and after looking into my eyes (iridology diagnosis) she asked me if she could bring Judith Collins in to see me. (Later Jayne told me there was nothing left in my eyes to see i.e. death.)

Jayne introduced Jack and I and started to talk to Judith, but Judith stopped her and said 'I know'. I lay on the healing table. Judith ran her hands over my body and immediately came back to the spot where I had the continual dull ache in my abdomen, although she had not been told anything.

She said 'My, that's deep — I will just lift that off there', as she began to hold her hands over the area for about ten minutes. The ache seemed to gradually go and never came back. Although I was still very weak, my life-force seemed to return to my body and from that day I gradually became strong.

That same evening I sat up at the dinner table and enjoyed my meal and am now healthy and happy. My husband Jack has always been a sceptic but after witnessing this miracle, he calls Judith 'Jesus Hands'. Whenever I have any health problems now, I visit Judith to keep me fit and healthy.

Margaret is one of the great doers of life! A retired nurse, she raised six children, developed and maintained an award-winning garden, all while working the long, arduous hours of a dairy farmer. A self-assertive, creative person, Margaret is also a very gifted potter. Her enthusiasm for life is contagious. When Brooke, her adolescent granddaughter, failed to gain pain relief from both doctors and natural health practitioners, Margaret implored the girl's mother to allow me to assess her. Just like her grandmother, Brooke was healed spontaneously.

Often people delay their healing process by putting off consulting me because of scepticism, religious beliefs or lack of belief. Here, Lee Gault tells her sorry yet happy tale of spontaneous healing. She was referred by her naturopath some eighteen months prior to seeing me.

Lee's story — Irritable bowel syndrome

I wish I had listened to the advice earlier. It may have saved me a lot of pain and disappointment as I can't thank Judith Collins enough for the help she gave me with the pain of irritable bowel syndrome.

Judith told me the healing would help unblock the problem. She held her hands over the crown of my head for a couple of minutes. I felt a sense of pulling to the top of my head as well as a numbing warmth. For my stomach, Judith held her hands over my lower stomach for a few minutes — there was a lot of gurgling and again a warm feeling. The pain was almost gone so I booked in for a second treatment. I felt great.

The process of healing was fantastic. After about four days I walked around feeling like I was 'off with the fairies'. I felt a sense of peace and serenity had come over me. Just to think 'no medication', just the touch of Judith's healing hands. It amazed me to realise that I had lived with this problem of stomach pain, bloating and excess wind for almost four years — after many trips to numerous specialists, naturopaths and medical doctors but to no avail.

I would recommend healing to anyone that is sick of being told there is nothing else that can be done to help them. I feel great and more at peace since my healing.

It makes you think that a lot more people could be helped by healing if they had an open mind.

CONVERTING RESISTANCE TO HEALING

There is no doubt in my mind that illness can become a habit. I find that a large number of my clients who have experienced their illness over a long period of time, experience difficulty in psychologically letting go of it. On awakening each morning they expect the pain or discomfort to present itself. This is a sign that the pattern is embedded in their consciousness. Commonly people also expect to suffer the diseases of their forebears.

To evaluate the hold an affliction has on you, listen to yourself to discover how often you use self-inhibiting language like this?

- My mother had it, so I *expect* I will end up the same way.
- It *runs* in the family.
- I can't walk too far because my legs *might* ache.
- I can't go to the concert because the loud music *might* bring on my headaches.
- If I eat that, it will *make me* sick.
- No matter what I do, I just *can't* lose weight.

Remember: bodily intelligence comes to accept restrictions and can form a stubborn resistance to change.

Those clients who heal relatively quickly don't appear to have a habit of using negative language. They say things like 'I can't wait to be rid of this; I've got so much to do' or 'I wish this would hurry up and heal' or 'I'm not spending my life being sick' — a much more positive approach. Rarely do they sink into self-pity or accept sympathy.

In order to encourage the healing of a disease you need to be 100 per cent certain that you want to get rid of your illness. You'd be surprised at how people hang on to an illness unconsciously because it either gets them attention, makes them feel wanted, brings the family back together again or gives them a way out of taking responsibility for their life.

I have found that when you have real purpose in your life you are more likely to be healed.

Three years ago a young woman came to me hanging her head as she tearfully described herself as having AIDS. The cause was a blood transfusion following the birth of her baby. As my heart cried out to help her, I said in a matter-of-fact manner 'So you've got AIDS. We'd best get to work and fix you'. I scanned her body and found several organs under attack. I suggested that we engage homoeopathy because of its wonderful reputation with this disorder. As I proceeded with the healing I spoke in a hopeful and healing tone. She talked incessantly of her new baby and her husband to whom she was clearly devoted.

Following several months of homoeopathy and two healing sessions with me, the debilitating effects of the disease had retreated. I never promised her a miracle, I simply offered her hope. That, together with her commitment, was enough to help turn what seemed like a hopeless situation into a ray of hope for a brighter future.

THE POWER OF HEALING CIRCLES

I developed the power to conduct healing circles some years ago. Since that time I have witnessed some wonderful spontaneous cures of conditions such as infertility, arthritis, asthma, migraine, back injury, chronic fatigue, Crohn's disease, hepatitis, and brain and heart disorders. I have come to understand that due to the unification of the healing energy, a healing circle is equivalent to three or four private healing sessions with me. A healing circle allows me to positively treat up to eighty people at the same time. I therefore value this means of treatment as it enables me to attend to the many people who seek me out.

In the healing circle, participants are seated closely together in a circle, with their hands clasped in a special way with those of their neighbours. The right hand faces upwards and the left hand faces downwards so as to allow the healing energy to flow rapidly and reach its maximum healing capacity. Eyes are closed to encourage relaxation.

As the group moves into a relaxed state of mind and body, I move behind each person in turn and lay my hands on their shoulders or head, allowing the healing to run into their body. The healing flows through their arms and links up via their neighbours' hands, thus flowing around the circle and building momentum.

The healing circle works at three levels: around the feet, directly flowing through the hands and in a warm band around the head.

SENSATIONS EXPERIENCED DURING A HEALING CIRCLE

Tingling in the hands and the feet is the sensation of the healing flowing through the body. However, when tingling is felt in the head or the body, it usually means that the healing is treating the blood, scarring or internal bruising.

Pulsing anywhere in the body indicates that the healing is addressing swelling, inflammation or internal growth.

Pain during a healing circle is the surfacing and the whole or partial release of a deep-rooted injury or ailment. It quickly rises to the surface and is released within minutes.

Pulling, drawing and **dragging** sensations are the adjustment of injury or illness. Intense drawing-out sensations can be felt in the treatment of cancer, heart and brain disorders, cysts, hernia and stomach and intestinal conditions.

A **jolt** in the physical body is often the adjustment of the skeletal body.

Hot and **cold** feelings are felt as blood pressure and body temperature adjust to a healthy medium.

A **cold spot** over the ailment often indicates stabilisation.

Localised piercing heat indicates that the healing is focused like a laser beam. This is common in the treatment of cellular disorders, and spine and joint disabilities.

A **warm embalming** sensation is a result of the body being saturated, from the head to the feet, in healing energy.

Excess body heat is the healing expelling toxins from the liver, kidneys, spleen, gall bladder, adrenals, pancreas and bladder.

Floating signals a shift in consciousness. As deep relaxation comes over the mind and body, a meditative state takes hold, allowing one to rise above the ailment and fully access the healing.

Lightness, a wonderful state of consciousness, indicates an emotional and physical adjustment. As most illness is the result of a deep-seated emotional disturbance, the feeling of lightness often precedes spontaneous healing.

Gurgling sensations and sounds can often be heard when the healing causes the digestive and intestinal areas to clear and/or regulate.

Momentary dizziness indicates an adjustment of the endocrine system.

Extreme heaviness is commonly felt as the muscles in the body are relaxed by the healing. As tension is released the sense of sinking into the weight of the body can at times be overwhelming but the outcome is wonderful.

No sense or **feeling** during a healing circle indicates that the person is either insensitive to their own feelings, resistant to relaxation or fearful of losing control.

It is impossible to participate in a healing service without experiencing something! Here Doreen, Sue and Jill wish to share their personal experience.

Doreen's story — Aneurism, neurological condition, lupus

I am a fifty-nine year old woman on an invalid pension and have suffered for over twenty years.

After having CAT scans and angiograms, a left internal carotid artery aneurism was discovered and diagnosed as inoperable.

Fifteen years ago I suffered a stroke, resulting in right-sided paralysis, and spent a year in rehabilitation at Shenton Park Hospital. Four years ago my head bleeds started. An attempted clipping and also embolisation with platinum coil was unsuccessful. This left me still with headaches and head bleeds, head tremors, eye drooping and more neurological problems after two brain surgeries.

In 1996 I attended Judith Collins' Healing Circle held in Perth. She touched my head three times and I have not had a headache or head bleed from that day. I have booked again for two healing circles and am confident that this time my lupus will be cured.

Thank-you Judith for sharing your God-given gift with me.

Sue's story — Neck and shoulder pain

As an interior designer, I have held a fascination for colour since I was given my first box of seventy-two Derwent colour pencils around the age of five.

More recently, reading Judith Collins' book *How to See and Read the Human Aura* gave me new insight into the way colour represents our emotions, feelings and thoughts. I could not resist asking Judith to draw my aura and of course the diagnosis was a remarkable reflection of myself.

I was also amongst the group of participants at Judith's Healing Circle. As we settled down joining hands, relaxing to the powerful music, Judith lightly touched each person in the circle for a few moments. We all received the gift of God's Divine healing flowing through Judith's hands. The energy was carried around the circle, conveying within moments a deep sense of relaxation, peace and ease. Without any physical adjustment, the muscular tension, nagging shoulder pains and jarring neck blocks melted away, leaving only a sense of lightness and gentleness. Thank-you Judith.

Jill's story — Heart condition

I had been an exhibitor at the *Mind, Body and Spirit Festival* in Melbourne for a few years and had seen Judith Collins' stand many times but had not had the time to see her personally. However, I was drawn to Judith.

In April 1997 I suffered a heart attack. In October of the same year, during a break from working at my stall, I sought her out. Judith was doing a healing circle at the show and a friend and I wanted to attend. But it was booked out. As we walked away from the booking office one of the staff called to us and said 'I have two cancellations'. We smiled at each other and thanked God and the Universe!

During the healing circle I felt tingling in my fingers and a deep, calm, relaxed feeling within. Following the healing circle I had more energy. My heart gave me less trouble and I was on less medication.

In January 1998 I had another relapse due to stress. A friend of mine, Cynthia, who often works on Judith's stall, informed me that Judith would be in Melbourne in March. On my behalf she telephoned and got me a private appointment. Following treatment, Judith suggested that I attend her healing circle the following evening. I experienced an incredible, powerful feeling. I felt embalmed in healing and energised. An hour later my left eye was irritated and started to swell. The flesh around the eye had turned black.

When I was a child and later as a teenager I was hit in the eye at a dance by mistake. I had to wear an eye patch for quite a while. Judith had warned all those in the healing circle that old injuries often surface so as to be healed. Undoubtedly but to my surprise I was evidence of this. My left side is weakest in my chest and it was my left eye that had turned black and swollen.

HOW TO HEAL LOVED ONES

The power of love is a wonderful healing tool. It encourages us to be compassionate and helpful to those who have earned our affection. When my mother once had a nasty fall due to a mild stroke, I implored the healing power to intensify. Being my best friend as well as my mother, there was no way I wanted to see her suffer. When I see this desire in others I take them under my wing and show them how to open to the healing power of love which is available to everyone.

A middle-aged woman brought her crippled and mentally retarded husband to me for healing. His injuries were sustained during a paralysing stroke which occurred whilst standing in a queue at the top of the stairs leading to a railway platform. He fell backwards, rolling down the stairs and onto the concrete platform. His injuries were extensive to say the least!

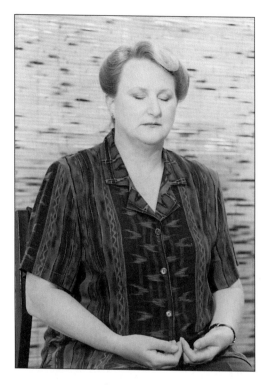

Attunement for healing

This position can be used to either prepare yourself to heal a friend or loved one or to gain access to the power of self-healing.

1 Set the atmosphere with music. Sit in a comfortable chair with your back in an upright position. Slouching causes a blockage in the flow of healing energy.

2 Turn the palms of both hands upwards so as to allow excess body heat or energy to release.

3 Close your eyes and relax your lips and jaw.

4 Through your nostrils take seven deep breaths, exhaling very, very slowly through the mouth.

5 Allow your breathing to become light and unnoticeable.

6 Repeat the healing invocation on page 57.

7 Relax. Feel the healing moving through your hands and body.

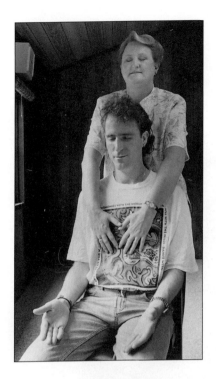

Stomach, liver and digestive system

Michael uses up his energy reserves and tenses his stomach and digestive tract when rehearsing and performing as a rock singer.

Here, my hands are clasped at the thumbs and at the index finger to ensure that the healing saturates the tension spots in his body.

He attunes to the healing by sitting upright with his hands turned upwards.

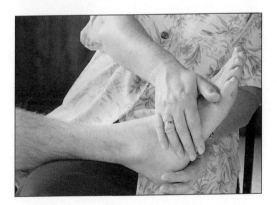

Ailments of the feet and poor circulation

Here, the foot is being cured of painful spurs which impair walking. One hand is placed on the heel and the other hand is held slightly above so as to remove pain and inflammation. This position can also be used to improve blood circulation in the legs and where joint damage has occurred.

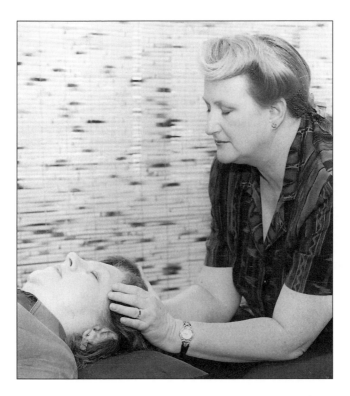

Core centre healing (blood/nervous/adrenal systems)

The nervous system, blood, endocrine and adrenal systems can all be treated using this position. Migraines too, respond to healing through this area of the body.

The patient is asked to close their eyes to help relax blood flow to the brain and nervous system.

To commence healing, place your hands slightly to the side of the head with the thumbs directly on the centre of the skull.

The patient may experience a build-up of pressure within the skull or a dizzy, floating sensation. Such feelings pass when the healing session is finished. Before walking the patient should sit upright for a few minutes so as to regain their sense of balance.

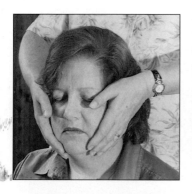 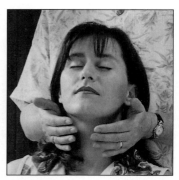

Treatment of facial and throat ailments

1   Roslyn is being treated for head tension which stems from her jaw being out of alignment, tension in the facial nerves and strained eyes.

    For treatment, hands are placed around and under the jawline and on the cheek-bone with the thumbs tucked under the eyes. This position can also be used for the treatment of hearing loss, imbalance, colds, and nasal and sleep disorders.

2   Libby is being treated for neuralgia as well as swollen glands caused by a virus.

    For treatment, the patient's head is tilted slightly back, resting on the healer's chest. The hands are placed under but away from the throat so as to release inflammation. The thumbs are turned upward toward the ears to allow the healing to flow to the head.

    This position can also be used for the treatment of weight problems, blood pressure, thyroid and parathyroid, vocal chords, lymph nodes, larynx and tonsillitis.

Eyes and brow

Hands are placed over and away from the brow with the fingers spreading over the eyes. In order to avoid head tension hold this position for three to six minutes only.

Eye diseases, addiction, allergies and the pineal gland can be treated using this position.

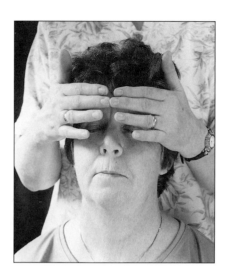

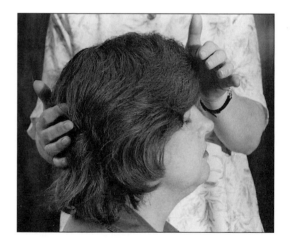

Migraine and hormonal balance

Head pain which stems from back, neck or hormonal problems can be treated by placing one hand firmly on the back of the head and the other hand above and away from the brow. The healing is channelled through the back of the head while pain and tension are released through the brow.

Menopausal hot flushes, infertility, memory loss, poor concentration, co-ordination and learning difficulties as well as hyperactivity can be treated using this position.

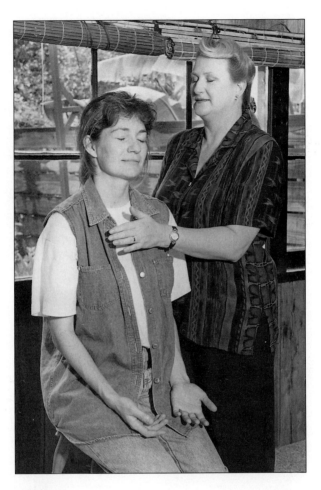

Treating asthma

Rebecca has suffered with asthma for most of her life. Here, she is being given relief from an attack.

1　She is seated in an upright position.

2　One hand is held on the back of the chest to send healing through to the lungs.

3　The other hand is held a few centimetres above the front of the chest to help draw out the congestion.

Rebecca's experience is one of warmth and calmness as you can see by the peaceful and contented look on her face.

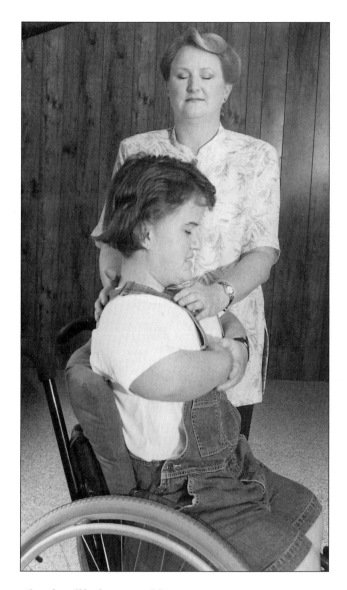

Strengthening life-force and immune system

Jocelyn is preparing to undergo intensive specialist surgery in the USA.

My hands are placed either side of the chest to reinforce her immune system and life-force as well as to alleviate anxiety.

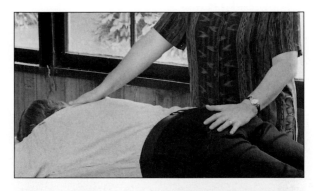

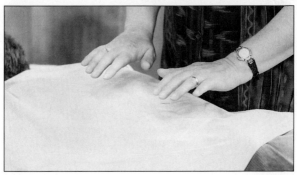

Back pain and injury

All types of back injury respond well to healing. The patient lies face down on the floor, a bed or massage table, with their arms beside them.

1 To remove stress and pain in the muscles around the spine, place one hand on their buttocks and the other hand between their shoulder blades, with your fingers close to the nape of the neck.

2 Spinal and disc deterioration is painful. More often than not, it cannot be touched. Hold both hands over the spinal region to draw out the pain and to help free-up movement in the area.

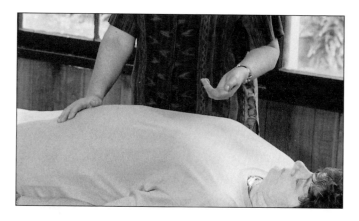

Drawing out inflammation and blockages

Barbara is receiving a treatment for menopausal complications as well as an imbalance in the bladder.

One hand is placed over the uterus and bladder region while the other is turned upwards and away from the body. This allows unwanted tension and aggravation to be drawn through one hand and out through the other. This position can also be used for the treatment of irritable bowel syndrome, relief of bowel and prostate cancer and to relieve pressure during pregnancy.

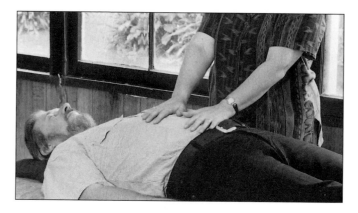

Stomach and bowel disorders

This position can be used to treat the trunk of the body for a large range of problems such as gastro-intestinal disease, nausea, heartburn, spleen, pancreas, gall bladder and bowel disorders.

Here, John is being treated for excessive gas which is causing the stomach to bloat. The healing will help to detoxify his body.

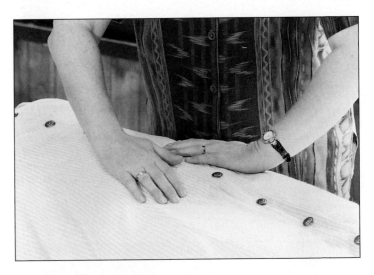

Treatment of the reproductive system

This position can be used to treat ovarian and prostate disorders, impotence, menstrual pain and irregularities, endometriosis, sexual problems, oestrogen imbalance, bladder infections, vaginal disorders, pelvic muscle cramps and hip joint problems.

The hands are placed lightly in the crest of the groin.

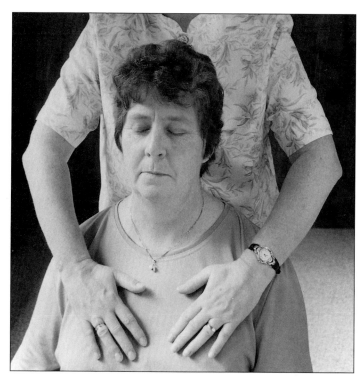

Breast cancer (breast/heart/lungs)

The position shown is for the treatment of conditions associated with the breast, heart and arteries, lungs and/or ribs.

Here, Irene has sought healing for a lump in her breast. Due to the ailment's slow receptivity to healing, I suggested she consult her doctor immediately.

His prognosis was removal of the breast.

Using this position prior to surgery, I was able to relax and prepare the area so as to ensure a speedy recovery.

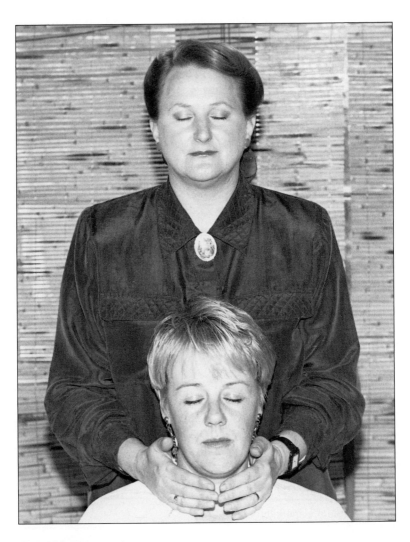

Thyroid cancer

Shawna McCoy of Camden, NSW, was healed of thyroid cancer in 1994 after several treatments. (Photo by John Appleyard.)

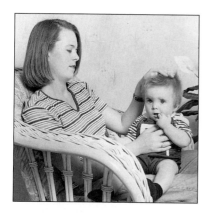 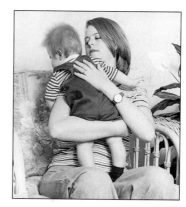

Healing an infant

Carolan is treating her son Ben for a few of the common ailments that afflict infants in their developmental years.

1   One hand is placed on his head to alleviate the trauma of teething. The other hand is spread over his digestive tract, stomach and bowel to alleviate nausea, reflux and loose bowel movements.

2   Ben is comfortably positioned over Carolan's shoulder so that she is able to spread her hand over the back trunk of the body to boost his immune system and life-force.

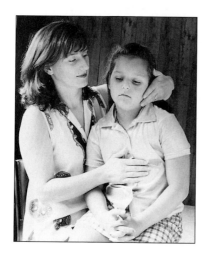

Treating childhood illness

Libby is treating her daughter Selina for ear-ache and nausea which has been caused by a virus. One hand over the ear and one hand over the stomach and pancreas will help to alleviate the child's discomfort.

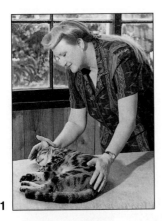
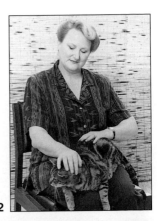

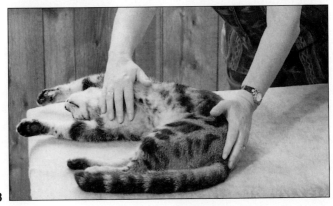

Animals

Animals that display a bond with their owner are receptive to healing. Here, we see my cat Barney posing for the camera. He loves spiritual healing.

After being bitten by a brown snake, he lost consciousness and became paralysed. The local vet could do nothing to help. He said that Barney's death would occur within a few hours and offered to put him down.

I was determined to heal him. And I did!

Healing was applied in all the positions shown.

1   Healing applied for the brain, blood and spine.
2   Healing applied for the ears, eyes, neck and bladder.
3   Healing applied for the digestive system.

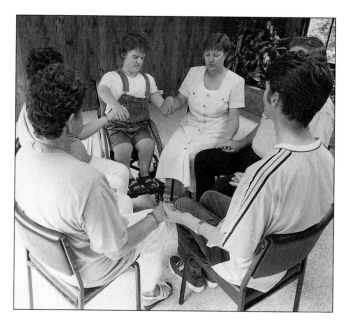

Family and friends healing circle

Jocelyn Powel suffers with complications associated with dwarfism. Here, family and friends seek to share their compassion and understanding by conducting a healing circle for her.

Seated in a circle, the group links hands with Jocelyn. The left palm faces downwards and the right palm faces upwards to encourage a smooth flow of energy.

Each member of the group focuses their thoughts on Jocelyn's disabilities and wishes for her well-being.

Music is played to relax the mind and body.

Spurred on by their contemplation and intention to heal, the circle will be saturated with healing energy after just twenty minutes.

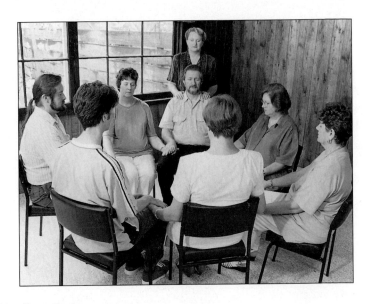

Healing circle

Participants gather in a circle for healing.

Seated with hands joined they prepare to allow the healing to transfer through their body and to their neighbours on either side.

I move behind each person placing my hands on their shoulders, head or in the centre of their back so that the healing has quick access to the body.

The healing flows down their arms and into their hands, spinning clockwise around the circle.

Participants are likely to feel tingling and warm sensations in their hands as well as a light feeling in the chest or head.

As the healing saturates their bodies and slows their metabolism, each person may feel tired.

The healing will continue to work through their system for approximately fourteen days.

Following the healing session I asked his wife how much she loved him. Her desperate tears answered, which was enough to convince me that her devotion could be used as a channel for Divine healing.

The healing exercise that follows, which I taught her and have shown many other people in similar situations, can be used by anyone who sincerely and devotedly loves or feels a deep compassion for the person who requires healing.

After twelve months of sharing this exercise, his wife's focused and loving healing had brought about his speech as well as the ability to feed himself and button his clothes — marvellous progress for a person so injured.

Healing exercise

Stand upright, with your legs slightly apart for balance and your knees slightly bent to reduce back and pelvic pressure. Place your hands gently on the shoulders of the patient. Take three deep breaths through the nostrils and exhale through the mouth very, very slowly. This helps to release tension and anxiety within the healer.

Once comfortable and relaxed, repeat this affirmation very slowly and sincerely until you feel a warmth flowing in and through the centre of the palms of the hands.

> The power of love is unconditional.
> It soothes and heals all who welcome it.
> I am/We are blessed with the power of love.
> Let the healing begin.

Allow the healing to run into the patient's body for ten to fifteen minutes only. If longer, the healer is likely to become drained and therefore be of little help to the ailing. Ten to fifteen minutes is plenty of time for the patient's body to become completely saturated in healing energy.

The photograph section in this chapter can be used as a guide to show where to place your hands for specific ailments.

GO WITH THE FLOW

As I previously pointed out, everyone has the ability to heal and nurture friends and relations. I believe it is our God-given right. We are charged with the responsibility to love and care for one another. Although spiritual healing is not meant to replace medical treatment it will no doubt enhance the well-being of the patient. And after every other option has been exhausted it is often all that is left to serve the sick.

One client of mine decided that she would learn to access her healing abilities in order to bring pain relief to her twenty-five year old son who had sustained serious injuries in a car accident. After six months of healing, her son was able to stand and walk. Two years later he resumed work as a landscape gardener. This was an amazing feat of love and commitment.

Some time later, my client was attending a presentation dinner with 300 other club members. Suddenly a member of the official committee had a heart attack. An ambulance was called. Without thinking, my client rushed to his aid, placed her hands on his chest and the healing flowed. By the time medical attention had arrived, his pain had ceased and his breathing was normal. He walked to the ambulance and was taken to hospital for assessment.

On her part, there was no premeditated thought. She simply healed with compassion and the healing flowed! A few weeks later the gentleman thanked her and described the sensations he experienced while receiving spiritual healing.

HOW OFTEN SHOULD YOU ACCESS HEALING?

I use one rule of thumb: *evaluate the effect of healing on the ailment*. Each person is unique and will respond differently. Some pain and illness can be stubborn and therefore requires the commitment of both healer and patient to see it through to relief or to a cure.

Some years ago I treated partial blindness in a man's eye. On the same day at the same time each week, he consulted me but with little result. I wanted to give up but he wouldn't let me. Then after sixteen treatments there was a breakthrough. Whilst getting into his car he caught a glimmer of light in the corner of his eye. Holding his hand over his good eye he realised that the blind eye was finally yielding to the healing. Nevertheless, he only regained partial sight in his blind eye.

There comes a time when one needs to recognise that even with our best intentions, and for whatever reasons, the patient will not be cured. It's a tough reality to face. One of my patients whose body is riddled with the pain of cancer, comes to me once every three weeks. Although doctors have prescribed the strongest possible pain-killers, occasionally the pain breaks through and she suffers terribly. Death parades itself on her face, yet lingers to taunt and to tease its beholder. She waits for that moment of release.

HELPING THE DYING

Healing, with its fine attunement to a Divine source, provides calm and solace to the dying. The focus of the healing is relief from pain and discomfort so as to achieve an inner peace, allowing one to let go of life as the time of death nears.

Exercise to alleviate pain and discomfort

1 A healer's hands should be placed on both the crown of the head and the chest, to facilitate a stillness within the patient.
2 Relief from pain and discomfort can be gained by placing the hands on or over the affected area.
3 During a hospital visit, healing can be channelled through the healer and into the body of the patient, simply by holding hands.

Some years ago I watched Donna Maberly, a young woman, walk the trail of death after having exhausted all conventional and natural treatments. Cancer was eating at her when we first met. But the two of us struck a chord and together we fought it tooth and nail for the sake of her, her husband and their children, one of school age and twins in infancy.

Donna left no stone unturned in her battle to nurture her babies. She subscribed to everything both orthodox and unorthodox. Riddled with pain and sometimes unable to make the slightest movement without discomfort, she undertook the arduous task to travel approximately 250 kilometres each week to consult me for healing. Together we turned a life expectancy of months into years. She had enough time to watch her babies grow into children; then she died.

During our final healing session she asked me what I would choose to have done with my body after it had died. I said I would be cremated and have my ashes tossed into the compost bin so that I would continue to be of service to the living planet, even when I'm dead, thus completing the circle of life.

Donna requested that people attending her funeral bring rose bushes to be planted in a circle with her ashes scattered about them in living memory.

A similar case comes to mind. Max Cuthbert was a man I came to greatly admire. He came to me seeking relief from bone cancer, arthritis and a pinched nerve. At first his response was excellent but a change in medication disrupted his whole metabolism and sent his recovery backwards. This made our job much harder. His resilience faltered. When he died, I wept bitterly. I knew we could have won the fight.

Both Donna and Max are etched in my memory as role models of personal strength in facing life's final challenge.

FAMILY AND FRIENDS HEALING CIRCLE

Healing can be enhanced by the coming together of family and friends whose compassion extends to the patient. The combined power of love can work wonders. It can ease pain, alleviate trauma and bring about relief and a cure.

Healing circle exercise

Sit in a circle, holding hands, with right palm upwards and left palm downwards, and eyes closed. Select a piece of music from the Recommended Listening list on page 127. I have tried and tested the effectiveness of this music to lift and focus a healing circle. It is essential to use music for relaxation and to help create a concerted effort. Take seven deep breaths through the nostrils and exhale through the mouth very, very slowly. Sit perfectly still.

Repeat in your mind several times.

> I am a vessel of Divine healing.
> With all my love I send to [name the person].

This affirmation encourages the healing to flow through the circle and into the patient for the duration of the healing circle (twenty to forty minutes).

When the patient is unable to attend

What happens when the patient is too sick or incapacitated to participate in the circle?

The circle is structured as indicated previously. Each person simply wishes the patient well. In this way, the power of the healing can be directed to the patient. This is called projected healing. It unites the power of love with the will-power of the mind, directing it wholly and solely to the patient.

HEALING AGAINST ALL ODDS

The world over, there are thousands of amazing stories of how people have cured themselves of the most horrendous ailments. The power of anointing with oil, baptising with holy water, prayer, self-realisation through meditation, and the magnetic power of love have all served to heal. I myself have witnessed what can only be described as miraculous. There appears to be no limit to what the power of the mind can achieve.

When I hear the term 'incurable' I think of all the people who have been relieved or cured either through my personal intervention or that of the natural health practitioners to whom I refer my clients. It makes me wonder what the term actually means. In many cases, the diagnosis 'incurable' frees a person to search and create a whole new journey.

This brings to mind a client of mine called Simon, who came to me to treat his shoulder injury. Whilst doing so, I noticed in his aura an old pattern of stomach cancer. When questioned, he told me the most remarkable story I had heard to date.

He was at work on a building site when a series of stomach pains caused him to lie in the foetal position for relief. Although having grown used to stomach pain, this time it was more intense. He could hardly move. A workmate bundled him into the car and rushed him to the local hospital.

Within an hour the pain was diagnosed as stomach cancer and an injection for pain relief administered. Anger rose in Simon's throat as the sentence of death 'three months to live' was proposed. He didn't hear what the doctor was saying. His mind was on his daughter who was that day sitting her Higher School Certificate exams. He also thought of his youngest daughter's dreams of one day cycling at the Olympics and lastly, the child who absorbed most of his attention, the daughter who was born deaf.

As he travelled back to the work site by taxi he could not engage in conversation. He stared at the photograph in his wallet of the woman he had loved for eighteen years. Repeatedly he asked himself 'How can I tell them? What will I say?'.

It was suggested by management that Simon spend the remainder of the day at home. In a quandary he drove around for an hour and then parked in a shopping bay. Wandering through the mall he found himself in a newsagency. A woman asked 'Can I help you?'. 'Not unless you can cure cancer' he replied. She ushered him along the aisle to look at half a dozen health magazines which offered natural treatment and pain management of disease. He bought three and returned to his car to read. With a mobile phone in hand he followed up a few advertisements and set about finding out what was available, all the while thinking that he had to have some hope to offer his wife and daughters.

Over dinner that night he explained to his family that the pain which his doctor had been treating was diagnosed as terminal. Before the tears of his loved-ones could flow he announced his plan. He had booked he and his wife into a macrobiotic cooking course so that he could immediately change to a healthy diet. He also enrolled them in courses of Tai Chi and transcendental meditation, to be followed by a ten-day meditation retreat in a month's time. He explained that he only had ninety days in which to cure himself — not because he had been told that he only had three months to live but because he had applied for and been granted three months long-service leave.

Simon and his wife walked together every day. The family laughed together every day too — this was part of the healing therapy. Gone were the television shows and videos that instilled negative values such as those that focused on dysfunctional relationships, fear, anxiety, violence and revenge. Only comedies were allowed. The whole family pulled together as they worked towards their goal. Eight weeks into the project, Simon awoke one morning with an overwhelming thought to have his progress medically assessed. 'All clear' was the diagnosis.

Months later, when I found the pattern of cancer, a look of shock came over him. I promptly explained that the etheric layer of the aura always shows what I call 'the scars of life'. That does not mean that an ailment will return in the future. No indeed! The etheric layer of the aura records life's experiences.

Every day somewhere in the world someone is being cured 'against all odds'. Countless clients of mine have walked away cured even though they have been told by the medical profession that their ailment is incurable. My own mother was told that she would have to live with a damaged nerve in her neck that far too often brought her to tears with its intense pain. Within two treatments of spiritual healing she was cured.

Harry Turner, a retired gentleman with a zest for life, came to a standstill when given the prognosis by his doctor. He shuffled about breathlessly and found even the most menial of tasks too strenuous. Doreen, his wife, came to tell me of his situation and explained that he would never agree to seeing a spiritual healer. But as fate would have it, the next client had cancelled their appointment. Doreen looked at me with an impish grin and asked if she could coax her husband into seeing me. He was sitting outside in the car. I'll never forget seeing this tall, stately man hunched over, monitoring every slow step he took. I'll let Harry finish the story.

Harry's story — Cardiac problems

I had been suffering from shortness of breath and a pain in the chest. A heart specialist informed me that my heart had an irregular beat. The associated breathing difficulties and painful digestive problem that was affecting the oesophagus were reducing my quality of life.

Since then I had been taking a tablet called Isoptin SR each day, having six-monthly check-ups and stress tests, and had been using a puffer for my breathing problem. The specialist informed me that I would have to live with my problem as there was no cure available. Ongoing medical tests, constant medication and the prospect of an operation on my oesophagus were not the reality that I wanted.

My wife, Doreen, had read an article in the local newspaper about Judith's work and decided that she wanted an appointment. I drove her to Earthkeepers and intended on staying in the car to read the newspaper. While there, Doreen asked Judith if she could treat my heart condition. Judith's affirmative reply prompted Doreen to call me from the car and with my permission I received the first healing treatment.

After two visits to Judith I felt my breathing becoming easier, my heart beat more regular and had a feeling of serenity. Judith concentrated on slowing down and regulating my heart beat. Subsequent treatments were directed to the oesophagus condition which has now 'calmed down' and is 'no problem'.

After my last six-monthly check-up, the heart specialist told me that my heartbeat is now normal and that I have the blood pressure of a twenty year old, not bad for a sixty-three year old. I now feel 100 per cent better than I was. Gone are the forty-winks-after-lunch syndrome!

Judith is something special — that something special in the lives of the many people she has helped.

When you have the best intention and a compassion to heal the sick, spiritual healing will open itself to you, whether through self-healing or when acting as a vessel for the healing of others.

Several of my clients agreed to be photographed so that others could see the hand positions I use for healing specific ailments. See the photograph section of this chapter.

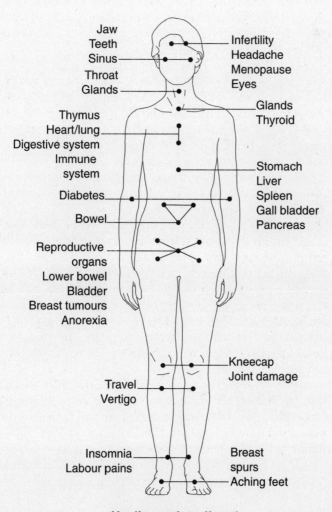

Jaw
Teeth
Sinus
Throat
Glands

Infertility
Headache
Menopause
Eyes

Glands
Thyroid

Thymus
Heart/lung
Digestive system
Immune
system

Stomach
Liver
Spleen
Gall bladder
Pancreas

Diabetes

Bowel

Reproductive
organs
Lower bowel
Bladder
Breast tumours
Anorexia

Kneecap
Joint damage

Travel
Vertigo

Insomnia
Labour pains

Breast
spurs
Aching feet

Healing points (front)

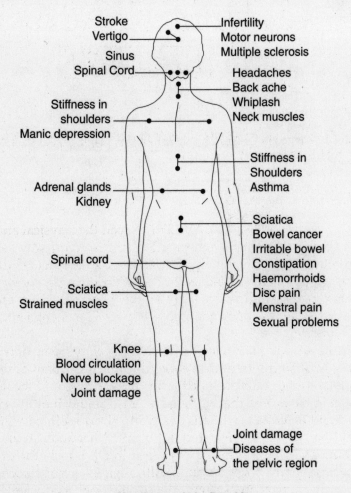

Stroke
Vertigo

Sinus
Spinal Cord

Stiffness in
shoulders
Manic depression

Adrenal glands
Kidney

Spinal cord

Sciatica
Strained muscles

Knee
Blood circulation
Nerve blockage
Joint damage

Infertility
Motor neurons
Multiple sclerosis

Headaches
Back ache
Whiplash
Neck muscles

Stiffness in
Shoulders
Asthma

Sciatica
Bowel cancer
Irritable bowel
Constipation
Haemorrhoids
Disc pain
Menstral pain
Sexual problems

Joint damage
Diseases of
the pelvic region

Healing points (back)

4 COMPLEMENTARY MEDICINE

RECOGNISING AND UNDERSTANDING AN AILMENT

MY ABILITY to read the physical and vital layers of the human aura allows me to frequently see clearly the cause of many physical, emotional and mental ailments as well as the side-effects of prescribed drugs, chemotherapy, radiation, biopsies and the like. However, there are times when illness does not clearly appear in a client's aura as a wound or disease.

While working at a show in Melbourne some years ago a young woman in her mid-twenties approached me to draw and analyse her aura for health purposes. All I could locate was an imbalance in the nervous system, a sluggish pituitary gland and hereditary patterns of arthritis. Disappointed with what I had to say, she abruptly interrupted my analysis and announced 'I have suffered with multiple sclerosis for the past three years'. I was stunned. Although aware of a problem with the nervous system, the seriousness was not evident. Her sister remarked: 'She looks wonderful doesn't she. There are no obvious signs. To look at her no one would even know. This is due to the strict regime of healthy living and meditation she adheres to'. I realised that with will-power and healthy living she was keeping the disease at a distance.

Further to this, in approximately one person in every hundred, the aura is so cluttered with the issues of life, that it creates a real challenge for me to specifically define or pinpoint disease. In these cases I am often heard uttering to my clients, 'God, help me. Where on Earth do I start?'. This is a sign of being overwhelmed. When unclear, I seek the assistance of professional natural and conventional medical practitioners.

Aware of the limitations of X-rays and biopsies, I am happy to use my abilities to assist the medical profession to locate the real source of complaint and avoid exploratory surgery. I believe in sparing the human body from the knife whenever possible. Most of my clients aren't too eager to be cut either.

Accurate diagnosis determines whether to use one or a series of specific treatments. Once I have located the 'cause' I assess the client's aura to see whether the healing process can be brought about sooner by incorporating other modalities. I assess the vibrational patterns in the physical layer of their aura to see if the ailment resonates to either acupuncture, homoeopathy, herbalism, osteopathy, chiropractic, shiatsu, aromatherapy, Bowen therapy, hypnotherapy, counselling or conventional medicine.

Kaye McClure, pleased with my assessment and advice, is happy to share her story of overcoming childlessness.

Kaye's story — Childlessness

I sought Judith's help as I had been trying to fall pregnant for nearly two years. I already had one son who was almost three by this stage (March/April 1995). I had been seeing a chiropractor on a regular basis for nearly a year and he was treating my pelvis which was 'out' and also sciatica in my legs (which I put down to continual aerobics). I had undergone a laparoscopy in February 1995 which basically found nothing wrong but had indicated that my left ovary was 'sluggish'. I was told this should not affect my fertility and to go home and keep on trying.

On the urging of mutual friends of Judith (John and Kate Puskas) I decided to seek her advice. At this stage I was willing to try anything and I was intrigued by a lot of what I had heard about Judith's abilities. When we met, she asked me why I wanted to see her. I only told her that I was trying to fall pregnant and wanted to know if there was anything that she could detect that was causing a problem. (I told her nothing about the chiropractor or the laparoscopy.)

She ran her hands over me, starting at the top of my head and moving down to my legs, stopping at several places to make comments. As her hands reached the back of my neck, she said that my pituitary gland was not working properly and would need some attention. When her hands reached my pelvis she said that my left ovary was blocked for some reason and was probably a big reason why I wasn't conceiving. She also said that my pelvis was 'out' and would need to be 'fixed up' before I could conceive successfully. As her hands continued down to my legs she also noted the pain in my legs from the sciatica.

When she had finished, she got down to the business of how I should go about healing myself. She gave me the number of a naturopath, Jayne Elder, who would be able to treat the problems with my pituitary gland and ovary. She said that two treatments of Bowen therapy would probably be all I would need to fix the problem with my pelvis and legs.

I came away from Judith's very excited that there was actually something I could do to help myself. I made an appointment with Jayne, who discovered quite a few problems with my 'system'. One of the main things I had to do was 'rehydrate' my inner organs by drinking two litres of water every day and giving up on caffeine in any form. I was also given a course of herbs and essences to begin the healing of my body. Jayne assured me that my problems were not too big and my body should be ready to conceive within three months.

I had two treatments (a week apart) of Bowen therapy with Carolan Nicholson at Earthkeepers Healing Sanctuary. I noticed after my second treatment that the pain in my legs had gone and I have not suffered with sciatica since.

I had another appointment with Jayne six weeks after my first visit and she said I was much improved. She wanted to see me in a further six weeks and felt that that would be all I would need. In fact, by the time I saw her at that third visit I was actually two weeks pregnant!!

I had a wonderful pregnancy helped along by Jayne's herbs and essences and some treatments with Carolan for headaches. I gave birth to Madeleine Anne on Good Friday, 5 April 1996, after an hour and forty minutes labour!

I truly believe that if I had not seen Judith when I did I would still have been trying today and probably would have gone through the trials of IVF. Not only do I have my baby, but I have also been exposed to a whole new world of healing and alternative methods of treating diseases and problems with the body. I am really deeply grateful to Judith for her perception of my problems and her solutions. That feeling that I could actually do something for myself was fantastic — as opposed to the advice given by doctors to 'just go home and wait'.

When all hope is taken from us despair sets in. Frequently I am able to direct people to the appropriate form of healing as well as a gifted practitioner, to bring about a more than satisfactory result.

A POWERFUL HEALING COMBINATION

I have noticed that homoeopathy and spiritual healing, when combined, can each increase the power of healing by up to eighty per cent. With this knowledge, whenever appropriate, I enlist the help of reputable homoeopaths such as Alan Jones of Chatswood and Lorraine Vine of Appin in NSW.

Lorraine Vine, whose practice is located twenty kilometres from my home and clinic, has in the past few years become my personal homoeopath. This is not just because she is within a comfortable travelling distance but is because of her giftedness, as well as her cautious yet enquiring mind, combined with a method of leaving no stone unturned in seeking an appropriate treatment. Because I recognise her abilities, I also refer my clients to her. I am particularly impressed by the way her prescribed homoeopathic remedies have reduced fluid retention in the lungs of my clients with liver cancer, emphysema and pneumonia. Homoeopathy allows the spiritual healing to concentrate purely on the cause of an ailment and not be distracted by complicated symptoms.

The combined healing power of homoeopathy and spiritual healing is described by Barbara Richards, a woman who I came to know and admire. Desperately ill and reduced to 'skin and bone', she mustered the energy to search for a cure.

Barbara's story — Digestive problems and general ill health

For years I had been feeling constantly unwell, as well as suffering from food allergies and digestive problems. Then, over a period of twelve months, I experienced a dramatic loss in weight and energy.

I sought help from GPs and specialists who put me through blood tests, X-rays, colonoscopies, ECGs, Scans, ultrasounds and faeces tests.

I heard about Judith Collins through my sister Joy, who was very much aware of my deterioration and whose little granddaughter was a patient of Judith.

My first visit was in November 1996. Judith found 'irregularities in the nervous system, thymus, pituitary gland, liver a bit sluggish and irregularities arising in the bowel'. This was frightening but it was a relief to at last have a diagnosis and to be offered treatment. I had a feeling of warmth from Judith's hands during healings and my health improved. On one occasion I was able to place my right hand under my left rib cage to feel a drawing sensation of something Judith was releasing. I not only felt but heard this release.

Although I'd made great improvement from the healings I could not stay well. A GP offered me anti-depressants which I accepted. Unfortunately this resulted in a complete physical collapse. On the day I travelled to return to Judith, a very dear friend who had sat with me until Kev arrived to make the journey with me, told me at a later date she did not think I would make it to where I was going!

Fortunately Judith was available for consultation and found 'blood disorders, sick blood, thymus malfunction and bowel and stomach problems'. I did not wish to return to doctors and welcomed Judith's referral to a colleague practising in homoeopathics, Alan Jones — a truly wonderful, remarkable man.

Using Judith's diagnosis, this very learned gentleman was able to explain that the problems were due to an overload of toxins in the liver—the result of long term stress, prescribed drugs and a diet containing sugars. He was able to treat me. This visit was the turning point for my return to good health. The initial treatment, detoxification of the liver, was horrific but with continuing homoeopathic treatments over five months there has been a ninety per cent recovery.

Thanks to Judith's diagnosis and Alan's treatment I have renewed energy and am well on the road to recovery. Without them I dread to think of my outcome. They are truly remarkable people. What a blessing to know such caring, friendly people. How unfortunate that alternative treatments are sought after all else fails. The human race needs re-educating. These wonderful alternative learned practitioners need to be heard.

I strongly believe that an energetic driving-force such as Barbara's can maintain a sense of self-empowerment and is a great advantage when tackling any illness. If I awake in the morning with a sore throat or stuffy nose I immediately take action to prevent it manifesting into something major.

Many people, however, think to themselves 'I'm a little worse than I was at nine o'clock and much worse than I was at eight o'clock'. Here, the mind is constantly focused on monitoring and encouraging the progress of the ailment.

COMPLEMENTARY MEDICINE

While working at the *Mind, Body and Spirit Festival* in Sydney during 1990, a large bushflower display attracted my attention. As I approached to examine it more closely, I saw tiny auric sparks of white, Delft-blue and gold light emanating from a display of brightly labelled bottles nearby. I was intrigued to learn how the bushflower essences were discovered and introduced by Ian White. We struck a chord and have worked together since that day. Ian has this to say.

Judith Collins has been a good friend and colleague and wise mentor to me for many years. During this time I have happily availed myself to receive healings from her. I consider Judith to be one of the foremost healers to be found anywhere.

On my first meeting with Judith, the thing that struck me most about her was her ability to instantly 'read' people; to know exactly what was happening and going on for an individual on all levels—emotional, physical and spiritual. All this she obtained by observing an individual's aura. I can assure you it is quite fascinating although a little unnerving to be 'seen so clearly'. Judith however tempers this gift with wisdom and insight, revealing to the individual only that which is sufficient to instigate a profound and catalytic effect within them. Her insights and interpretations of the aura are extremely powerful, knowledgeable, accurate and clear.

Having witnessed her visionary healing around the world, whether one-to-one, or with groups, I totally recommend Judith and her tremendous work to you.

AUSTRALIAN BUSHFLOWER ESSENCES

These homoeopathic drops play an integral role in healing the mind, body and spirit. Conventional medication, while eradicating most symptoms, does not always address the cause. Furthermore, side effects can be seen in the aura for many years, clogging systems and causing a sluggish response in organs, especially the pancreas, liver and kidneys.

It didn't take me long to realise that bushflower essences (some more than others) perform well in conjunction with my healing work. Consequently, numerous essence bottles line the shelves of my clinic's dispensary. I frequently refer to the essences. I simply glance at my client's aura, then scan the dispensary shelves using the etheric energy of my left hand to match their auric vibrations. This system of reference has fascinated Ian for years, not only because I always choose what he himself would prescribe but also because I have been able to describe to him additional healing potentiality of a number of essences.

I regularly use the following essences in conjunction with my healing sessions because of their ability to blend with the healing vibrations. In fact, I have noticed that when you combine homoeopathic remedies with spiritual healing, the response to healing is increased.

Dynamis gives a subtle yet noticeable lift to petering energy thus leaving the person feeling revitalised. I have found it of value to those suffering with tiredness, physical exhaustion and chronic fatigue.

Confid balances thought and emotion to produce confidence and self-empowerment.

A middle-aged businessman who found himself unemployed suddenly developed panic attacks whenever he applied for a new job. I suggested he use Confid to help overcome his nervousness. After three days he found that the panic attacks had reduced and that the confidence he needed to regain work was slowly but surely increasing.

Cognis creates a greater unification of the mind and the body, which in turn leads to increased concentration and focus.

My mother, who was noticing distortion of her memory, asked me to help prevent the deterioration. This essence worked slowly but surely. I now recommend it to all my ageing clients as well as menopausal women, slow learners and nervous students facing exams.

Heartsong encourages greater self-expression and helps to overcome shyness and inner fear. I recommend it to all those applying for new jobs, auditioning for the theatre or about to engage in public speaking or debate.

A young man who had planned to defend himself in court against traffic offences was aware that he often became tongue-tied when nervous. After taking the essence for only one week prior to the event he celebrated his eloquent defence.

Travel can prevent travel sickness and alleviate vertigo.

I love this essence because it prevents me from suffering jetlag as I fly from coast to coast or country to country. It's wonderful to have in the glove box of the car. At the first sign of anyone feeling sick or dizzy, place seven drops under their tongue and they are well on the way to recovery.

Solaris aids in the healing of burns. It brings to the surface old sunburn damage. One young woman took it to help combat side-effects from radiation treatment of her cancer. Within days a five-year-old bikini sunburn line surfaced.

A man grew tired of having skin cancers cut out every few years. He decided to bring them all to the surface by taking Solaris to ascertain the real problem. To his astonishment within five days of taking the drops his face was pink and red from skin cancers which had surfaced. He was now able to take affirmative action.

Emergency is always in my handbag. It causes the body to come into alignment. Therefore floating germs and viruses are easily eradicated before they really take hold. At the first sign of a sore throat, blocked nasal passages or head tension due to a long and tiring schedule, I place a few drops under my tongue and I quickly bounce back to good health.

Relationship helps to untangle trying and non-communicative relationships, creating a degree of harmony. A concerned mother did not know what to do with her six-year old twins who verbally and physically fought day and night. After the girls took the drops for one week, harmony began to appear. Three weeks into the medication, the girls had reached a tolerance of each other.

Meditation encourages receptivity to spiritual and intuitive vibrations. I recommend this essence to all my clients who find it difficult to unwind at the end of a working day and to all the chronically ill clients who must relax in order to heal themselves.

BOWEN THERAPY

Bowen therapy was developed in Geelong, Victoria, by the late Tom Bowen. It is now taught worldwide and is perhaps the modality that impresses me most. Its gentle touch on soft tissue stimulates the body's energy flow, empowering itself to heal. One simple movement sends changes rippling through the body. A stiff neck can be released within minutes. Menstrual pain can be dissolved within minutes too. Its speed of corrective treatment of physical restrictions such as tennis elbow and frozen shoulder are quite remarkable. Fortunately I am married to one of the best Bowen practitioners in Australia and have the chance to be treated regularly. Paul's unique approach has won the respect of professional sports people and accident victims.

HOMOEOPATHY

Homoeopathy calls on the body's own substantial reserves to heal itself. In theory it is fundamentally different to established medical practice because of its philosophy that 'like can cure like'. In other words, a substance which can produce symptoms in large doses can cure similar symptoms in minute doses. For example, if taken in excess, May Apple causes profuse and foul-smelling diarrhoea. But in a homoeopathic preparation it is called podophyllum and is used to cure the same symptoms.

A homoeopath uses a potentising machine to create dosages so minute that not a single molecule of the original substance can be detected in the medicine. Potentising is a system of dilution and succussion which releases the energy of the original substance. Several drops of this tasteless remedy under the tongue can take effect almost immediately.

Over fifteen years ago I consulted well known homoeopath Alan Jones of Sydney, to heal my allergic reaction to smoke. This affliction not only clogged my breathing apparatus, it also produced painful sores in the nostrils. Alan prescribed a homoeopathic remedy and said that the allergy would subside in about two weeks. However, unbeknown to me at the time, my aura resonated strongly with homoeopathy and so I was cured within four days.

When a practitioner makes an accurate diagnosis, as seen in my own case, ill health can vanish almost spontaneously. It vibrates to the very essence of our life-force and so can have a powerful impact.

ACUPUNCTURE

Acupuncture is recognised as the world's oldest medical system, dating back over 2000 years. It was brought from China to western society during the 17th century by Jesuit priests. It works with the flow of 'chi', a subtle energy that flows through fourteen clearly defined channels known as meridians in the human body. Thin needles are inserted at specific meridian points to regulate the body's flow of energy. It also fascinates me because long after the needles have been removed, chakras and meridians display the healing effects. I have noticed that acupuncture is particularly effective with stroke victims.

My mother suffered a mild stroke which left her partially disabled. Her doctors prescribed physiotherapy but it failed her. My father suggested chiropractic treatment but it too failed her. On my return from an interstate lecture tour I assessed her aura and announced that acupuncture was the key. After only eight treatments my mother was completely cured.

THERAPEUTIC AROMATHERAPY

Therapeutic aromatherapy is the application of essential oils to open the body to healing through stimulating its senses. Jasmine uplifts. Yarrow soothes. Essential oils represent the soul of the plant from which they are extracted. They are the most concentrated form of herbal energy and have powerful antiseptic, antibiotic and antiviral properties. They are used externally in the gentle process of aromatherapy massage and through inhalations.

My husband Paul, a highly respected aromatherapist, combines essential oils for localised application by his clients. He has a blend of oil to alleviate cramps and to facilitate muscular strain during childbirth, a blend to relieve skeletal pain, a blend to release muscular tension and to release pent up stress, a blend to relieve varicose veins . . . the list seems endless. When the family is choked up with the flu virus, he burns lavender oil, a decongestant to clear the breathing passages and to aid sleep. Five drops of rosemary oil is added to warm bath water to soak tired and strained muscles.

WORKING WITH DOCTORS

'What do the doctors think of you?' asked a client. 'Well', said I, 'some love me, some think I am a charlatan, some regularly refer their clients, some engage me to professionally work by their side, some have attended my healing classes and some come to me for personal treatment'. The one thing they have in common is a need for privacy due to professional prejudice. Therefore for ethical reasons Dr David G. of Brisbane, Queensland, while enthusiastic in sharing his own story, must remain anonymous.

Dr David's story — Judith's clairvoyance

The Epistle to the Hebrews, Chapter 13, verse 2, reads: 'Do not forget to entertain strangers, for by so doing some have unwittingly entertained angels'.

Judith Collins does not pretend to be an angel, but in the minds of many people she is all that and more. From her earliest years, Judith has been acutely aware of her ability to sense and see the aura, which is invisible to most people. But this reflection of the life-force that gives both the dimension and direction of energy fields, Judith acknowledges as a Divine gift and blessing.

In November 1995, in the middle of what has been described by others as 'the dark night of the soul', I was introduced to Judith at a *Health and Harmony* symposium. She came up to me in the small crowd, took me by the hands, looked at me with penetrating eyes and said 'You must be a doctor — certainly a healer. Please come and see me after this session'. Apprehensive and bewildered, I sought her out and found her sitting with her husband.

Judith told me that I was in the process of acquiring immense knowledge, that I was embarking on a huge new venture and that I had incredible energy and stamina. She also said that although I was in excellent health, I would experience much congestion in my upper respiratory tract and bronchial tree. Judith told me other things which are too personal to share about the past, present and future. Above all else, she urged me to be strong, courageous and patient and told me all would be well.

The fact was, I was about to leave on an extended overseas trip to research hyperthermic oncology and bio-immunotherapy. Furthermore I was committed in a joint venture business to build a clinic in the same field, and had a debt of more than $1 million. Faced with the derision, opposition and scepticism of medical colleagues and 'friends', my encounter with Judith proved timely.

The research project went exactly as planned, only it was far more enriching and fulfilling than expected. I met the right people at the right time in the right place. It was unbelievable—an assembly of the world's leading medical scientists and specialists who represented the very best in state-of-the-art oncology. However, right in the middle of the Scandinavian winter I contracted a severe head and chest infection. Not having been sick for many years, it took me by surprise. Then I remembered Judith's prediction.

About a year later I met Judith again. She said: 'You are going very well, aren't you? But I see a big problem in a few weeks with authority'. She said it could be the city council or another figure or organisation of authority.

Naturally I was concerned. She predicted it would last several months but that it would not be devastating. She said that it would start about 5 December! Right on target, a letter arrived that very day from a federal government depart- ment. It later proved to be a total mistake but it cost me thou- sands of dollars. Exactly one week later, 12 December, while interceding for a special friend who was seeking a visa to visit Australia, I struck a total impasse!

Three months prior, Judith had said on the telephone that she believed that things would start to move very well on about the 14th of the month. Once again, as if right on cue, an incredible sequence of life-changing events started rolling forward very positively.

Over the years, Judith has, with her Divine anointing, pin- pointed and described very accurately, disease processes in many patients that I have referred to her for counsel. Judith Collins, healer and seer, continues her humble work — bless- ing and strengthening all those privileged to cross her path.

Working with both orthodox and natural health practition- ers interests me greatly. Wherever I work in this country and overseas I build up my resources and seek out reputable services from those purporting to be healers. The types of prac- titioners to whom I refer clients have to display a natural flair for their profession. In this way I know that my clients are get- ting the best possible service. Too often, the people who seek out my service have already done the rounds of GPs, hospitals, naturopaths, chiropractors and the like. I need to be certain that I am working with the best so that clients are not let down again and to ensure quality of healing.

A client asked me to visit a severely injured relative in hos- pital. The patient was unconscious and in an intensive care unit. In front of two doctors and three nurses I nervously scanned his body and commenced the healing. I could feel their scepticism and attempts to erode my confidence. The defi- ant nature of my adolescence returned to me momentarily to provide protection. When I began to announce my findings, his relatives gathered round and listened with fixed attention. The medical crew, however, listened half-heartedly. On my return to the hospital two days later, my findings had been medically confirmed.

5

PERSONAL HEALING JOURNEYS

Lyn's story — Arthritis

I HAD SUFFERED pain and swelling in my right knee for many years, trying all sorts of remedies ranging from the old washing-soda-overnight trick to creams to lotions to physiotherapy — you name it. I had even had an arthroscopy where the surgeon trimmed the cartilage and tried to clean up some arthritis which he found in the joint. In addition, after trying all sorts of diets, I had discovered a low fat regime which, coupled with 25 minutes of power-walking three times a week, was resulting in weight loss — feeling good! However, the walking began to aggravate the knee so much that it ballooned each time I exercised and gave me great pain. I saw an arthrologist who gave me eight cortisone injections over a lengthy period, as well as taking fluid off the joint using aspiration. As a fully-paid up wimp, this did not please me at all! The last try was an injection of yttrium in the knee at Monash Medical Centre and a week off work to keep the joint still. Sadly, this did not work either.

I had resigned myself to a life of pain and discomfort, and life wasn't all that bright and cheery when Judith happened to come to the office to discuss a forthcoming book. This was just before the *Mind, Body and Spirit Festival* at the Exhibition Centre in 1997. Some of the editors and the Marketing people were in the boardroom with Judith and Paul, and in the course of the conversation my name came up with the suggestion that I should come along to the Show and get some help. Judith immediately said 'Oh, bring her along now!'. So suddenly, much to my surprise, I was whisked away from my computer, down to the boardroom and told to sit down as Judith would do some healing on my knee.

I sat down and went to show Judith where the problem was. 'I don't need to see the knee', she said, and placed her hands on either side of the balloon and went on chatting to me, Paul and the other people in the room. I was at a bit of a loss, as not only was this quite unexpected but I had imagined a hush, and soft music and a definite ambience! I couldn't get over the heat of Judith's hands, and when she moved her hands, it was the absence of heat which was the most noticeable feeling. A couple of minutes into the session, Judith said 'Ah, there was just a little adjustment of the bone there' although I couldn't feel any sensation. I have no idea how long the session lasted, I just sat there in the middle of all this activity feeling quite at sea. Finally Judith removed her hands and asked me how that felt. I felt fine, and said so, hoping that this would last. You tend to get a bit dispirited after you feel you've tried everything. Judith remarked that I should give myself a bit of time off that evening, which I took to mean, 'don't do the ironing after dinner'! I walked away from the boardroom quite comfortably, feeling that I'd like to think this was going to work.

After dinner, as suggested, I sat down to 'veg out' in front of the TV. When I awoke an hour later, the family suggested I would be better off in bed rather than out like a light in the chair, so I tottered off to bed at 8:45 pm. I lead a very busy life, and this was most out of character for me. It was an even more out of character occurrence to wake up at 10:00 am the next morning! I had seemingly hit a brick wall. Judith explained later that the treatment had extended to every cell in my body, each and every one in need of R & R after having had the arthroscopy.

I had another two sessions while Judith was in Melbourne. (She gave me the first session at no charge, for which I am most grateful. We had had to suspend our health insurance, and after all those treatments there was very little money left in the kitty!) In addition, Paul promised to send me some of his arthritis oil which was one of his aromatherapy treatments.

Little by little my knee began to settle down, and pain began to subside. I was still having to sleep with a small pillow under the knee, as the angle of the leg during the night was crucial. However, I started to get a little more sleep as the pain became less severe. A reasonable night's sleep is very precious!

Barbara's story — Back injury

In 1990, I injured my back (ruptured disc) at work and since that time I have consulted many physicians for relief from the constant pain and discomfort. After the injury I was admitted to hospital for traction for three weeks and then had to take three months off work to try and get back to a reasonable state of health. I also tried acupuncture, physiotherapy, periodic traction and swimming exercises, all to no avail. I have struggled through the past seven years in constant discomfort and have had to do all the menial tasks of just living, for example, gardening, ironing, housework and employment — in pain.

Since being treated by Judith Collins, I have had great relief as far as my back is concerned. I am now able to do my housework without feeling pain whilst doing it and also for the rest of the day. I can now move much more easily, to the extent that I can almost say, with very little discomfort. I did however feel a lot of discomfort for a couple of days after the healing — a dragging sensation around the lower back and lower stomach area. I also felt something move within my back whilst sitting one night at home in my armchair. It felt like a muscle or tendon moved to the right — a strange sensation and one that I had never experienced before. I was also experiencing severe stress and tension pain in the upper part of my back/neck. My neck was very stiff and painful to move and I had difficulty in turning my head from side to side. Since having just two healing sessions, I now am able to move my neck with very little pain. It still cracks but this I believe is due to degeneration of the vertebrae and is something that cannot be cured.

I had never contacted anybody like Judith Collins before and I guess I was a little sceptical. But after being given a magazine at the local railway station which featured training courses and so on, and seeing an article on Judith's healing, I plucked up the courage to contact her and make an appointment. I was really desperate and frustrated at the time and was searching for help to enable me just to get to work and perform my job comfortably, and without pain.

I am now able to do this and have felt generally that I can walk and move around with much more ease. For this I have Judith to thank and look forward to continuing to have a life without too much pain. I still have two more sessions to attend and therefore expect that my condition will improve even more. I would like to say that anyone with health problems should at least take the time to visit Judith Collins and try her methods of healing. I can recommend it.

Sue's story — Childlessness

After three years of tests, surgery and being on a fertility programme, my husband and I were about to give up on ever having a baby of our own. Then, after reading an article about Judith and how she has helped so many with her spiritual healing I decided to see her. To be honest I did not believe in spiritual healing, but we were so desperate to try anything and I felt I had nothing to lose.

On my first visit to Judith, she was able to tell me exactly what was wrong and she began to work on 'healing' the problem. After only my second healing session with Judith, I found out that I was pregnant. I was so delighted and amazed.

Last year I gave birth to a beautiful, healthy baby girl. I had a totally natural birth without any drugs. The labour was only 2 hours 30 minutes!

I will always be very grateful to Judith. She is an amazing woman with a very special gift.

Adam's story — Electrocution

This is my story of electrocution, which occurred during a school term break in the year I was sitting my School Certificate at the age of 15 years, and the treatment and healing that I have experienced since that event.

On a nice warm sunny Sunday afternoon of 7 July 1996, I was cleaning the car. As the cord for the vacuum cleaner was not long enough to reach from the power point to the car, an extension cord was required.

As I was plugging one extension cord into the other, the ring finger of my left hand slipped in between and onto the prong of the cord. The power grabbed me and I started to feel a weird sensation jolting through me. I fell to the ground and tried to pull my hand free but was unable to do so. I screamed out 'Mum' a few times as my left arm and right leg started to shake uncontrollably.

Mum came running out as she sensed and heard the fear in my voice and saw me attached to the power cord. She raced inside and switched off all the power cords plugged in near the doorway. She came out to find me still attached and yelling out 'The bedroom, the bedroom'. She then ripped the fly screen off the window, leaned in through the open metal window frame and pulled the power cord from the power point as she couldn't reach the switch.

With the power supply disconnected, I was then able to free my hands from the cord. I immediately stood up and grabbed my left arm just above the wrist, and the hand where I felt immense pain. I also told Mum I wasn't going to the hospital. After asking me how I was, Mum looked at my hand and said we were going to the hospital immediately and that it was not negotiable. I put on my shoes whilst Mum looked for her car keys. She drove me to the Emergency section of the nearest hospital, asking how I was going, if I was in much pain and keeping a general eye on me. I had a very deep hole in both my ring finger and tall man and a burn mark on the side of my little finger but no hole and I was unable to straighten my third and fourth fingers. I wondered if it was the actual bone I was seeing on the two fingers when I looked at the damage.

Luckily at Emergency there was only one person waiting at the reception desk. We gave my particulars and were told to take a seat in the waiting area. No sooner had we taken our seats when my name was called by the triage nurse and off we went to her room. She asked what I was there for and I told her 'electrical burns to my hand'. She asked if we were talking electrocution, to which I replied 'yes'. I didn't even get to sit down and here she was whisking me out the back door of the room, down the corridor and into some other area. I was given a hospital gown and told to take off all my clothes, change into the gown and get up on the bed immediately.

No sooner had she left, than a male nurse came in and hooked me up to a machine that monitors the heart, pulse, blood pressure and whatever else. Talk about your worst nightmare — I had just been electrocuted and they were hooking me up to electrical machines.

A doctor came in to check me over. Much disagreement arose over the entry and exit points of the electrical current — these need to be established in the treatment of electrocution burns. I was checked from head to toe for the exit point but they were unable to find it. Mum asked if it was possible for the entry and exit points to be in the fingers, to which she was told they felt not.

The doctor commented on how my heart was pumping like a choo choo train and asked me how the injury occurred. When I told her, she replied with 'Lord save me from teenagers and their stupid pranks', which was very esteem shattering. She informed us that I was to be admitted to a hospital but that she needed to make a few phone calls before she could tell us where. I told Mum I didn't want to stay in hospital, that I wanted to go home and right now.

Talk about being a display showpiece. The medical personnel on duty at the time came from all over the hospital just to see my burns as they don't get much opportunity to see such good and deep burns. I wasn't even asked if I minded.

The doctor came back to tell me that I was being transferred to another hospital, that I would be admitted there as it was a trauma hospital and that an ambulance would arrive shortly to transport me. I would probably be in theatre before the night was out. They wouldn't even allow me to use the bathroom as I had to remain hooked up to the machine at all times. My hand was washed with saline solution, covered with a cream, enclosed in a sterile bag that was sealed around my wrist and a catheter inserted into the back of my right hand.

The ambulance arrived. After retelling of the incident, I was transported to the next hospital, where I was again hooked up to a machine. The blood tests that the admitting doctor had requested had not been done by the first hospital, so they drew my blood and didn't even use the catheter.

What a waste of a pinprick. A drip was started so as to build up my body fluids as I was required to give another specimen. I graciously gave my blood to the drip every time the machine took my blood pressure, which the hospital staff didn't seem to appreciate very much.

I was finally admitted near midnight and was not to be operated on that night after all — it would probably be in the morning. I was seen the next morning on rounds by the plastics registrar and whoever else, and informed that I would probably be operated on later, once the consulting specialist had seen me.

The physiotherapist Greg was the next person I saw. He made a prosthesis hand/wrist support for my left arm which could be taken on and off, and gave me exercises to do. My hand was still covered with a dressing that was changed each morning, and enclosed in a sterile bag. Eating meals was a classic with a catheter in one hand while the other hand was in a sterile bag supported by a prosthesis. The meals didn't arrive cut up for me.

The consultant specialist plastics that I had been admitted under, didn't show until Wednesday evening. He told me that a full-thickness skin graft would be performed on my fingers. The doctor, like the registrar, was amazed and astounded at how much function I had been able to get back into my fingers since my injury. After such a long wait, the catheter was removed from my hand.

It helped that Mum had spoken with me about the accident before I went in to theatre. She let me know that as a mother her natural instinct was to protect but that she was not God and couldn't possibly be everywhere; nor could she have protected me from this accident or change the pain I was now suffering. She said if she could change places with me she would but that it was not possible. She told me that what she had done to disconnect me from the power was more stupid than anything I had done and that she could have created more problems than there were already. What had happened to me was a freak accident. People plug in and disconnect cords from power points that are left on all the time. Mum felt I had a purpose in life that hadn't been fulfilled yet and that I was a walking miracle. She told me not to let other people pull me down by suggesting it was a stupid teenage prank because I knew, like she knew, that it wasn't.

I was amazed to learn whilst I was in hospital, just how some people had been electrocuted but not suffered anywhere near as severe burns. Most were thrown by the electricity whereas I was grabbed by it. One was electrocuted when putting Christmas lights on a Christmas tree. Another was electrocuted by a tape player that had been left outside before it rained. When she went to pick it up, she was thrown by the electricity. Another was working outside with electrical power when one of his children decided to be helpful, turning on the power inside and the father being electrocuted. He even showed me the resultant graft work and donor site used for what was done many years before. His only disability was that he did not always feel what he was holding, thus dropping things because he had lost the sense of touch. Some people told me they plug cords in and out of power points with the switch on, even when their partners go crook at them. Another suffered burns when a hair drier blew up in her hands whilst she was using it. I learned that an ELCB (earth leakage circuit breaker) would not have helped me in this instance as it had not helped the people in the above situations who did have ELCBs on their circuits. Many people touched me during my stay in hospital.

The operation was performed on Friday afternoon of 12 July by the plastics registrar. He will be a very much sought-after specialist one day. The donor site for the skin graft was my upper inside left arm. Two miniature pins (like tent pegs) were inserted into my fingers, to straighten them out. As I was in pain when I returned to the ward, I was given some pain killers. As fast as these hit my stomach, they were brought up again and the bed covers and clothes changed.

I was discharged the next day with my instructions and an appointment to see the plastics registrar in emergency the following Thursday to have the dressing taken down and the pins removed. I was given a week off school.

Even though I like blood and guts like a typical teenager, the removing of those two pins in my fingers was even too much for me. I almost fainted. I was laid down and instructed to take deep breaths in the hope of not leaving an unwanted present. I was given an appointment to see a physio the following morning. It was my friend Greg from when I was in hospital. Well, these sessions started with much pain and agony. I think we were both fortunate to have a table in between us at the sessions. Greg was most frustrated at not being able to work out when I was in pain and when I wasn't, as I was quite uncomplaining and unyielding.

Monday saw my return to school for only five minutes because no sooner had I arrived than I was on my way up to sick bay. My hand was pouring blood through all the bandages like a tap had been turned on. I met Mum near the entry to the office. She hadn't yet left the school since she was speaking with my year coordinator. Needless to say it was an immediate trip back to the hospital. The doctor took down the dressing and thought that the grafts were still good.

Only one further bleed out occurred that week. However, I was to learn the following Monday after seeing the admitting consultant specialist plastics that both grafts had failed. I'm not sure who was the most disappointed, me or the plastics registrar who had performed the surgery.

The following Friday I had another graft. Ten days later I was told that the graft on the tall man was alright but that the one on the ring finger had failed. I couldn't believe it — another failed graft, and so fast.

The following week the admitting doctor told me that nothing further would be done. They would wait and see what eventuated over the next twelve months as age was on my side and to determine my disability and what needed to be done. Mum was jumping up and down with that remark.

Over the next few months I continued with Outpatients, physiotherapy and monitoring by the community nurse. Progress was slow. Surgery was again considered but both Mum and I were against this.

Mum arranged for me to see some other specialists who were located some distance away. Nothing very positive was forthcoming. I was advised to live with my disability and learn to work around it as other people do. It was suggested that I become more academic: since my hand was affected, it would be a handicap to me in most trades. It was also recommended that it was about time Mum let go of the apron strings. My immediate thought was that I would get the full use of my hand whatever it took and that I would prove these doctors wrong. I figured I was determined and stubborn enough to prove it to everyone.

Mum began to spend many hours using her knowledge of Chinese massage, for which she holds certificates, as she tried to relieve the pain in my left wrist and arm. She also used her knowledge of sound vibrations using a Tibetan bell and singing bowl which helped close the wound to my fingers. At this point she began to investigate alternative healing methods of a variety of practitioners.

One day Mum received a flier in the mail for courses with Judith Collins that were being held at Earthkeepers. Mum had met Judith during the *Mind, Body and Spirit Festival* at Darling Harbour in May 1996. How they met is a story of its own. Also, Mum had been wanting to attend Judith's course on the Human Aura for some time. She did this on 22 February 1997. She learnt more about Judith and her work whilst at the course. She spoke to me about this when she returned home. One thing led to another and next thing Mum was asking Judith if she could possibly help me or advise what type of therapy might be of assistance to me.

I met Judith for the first time on 19 March 1997 and received spiritual healing. Of course I am not one for doing anything that involves pain and I let her know. Judith informed me that neither was she. That was very comforting to know. I lay on the table and felt nothing. Judith asked if I could feel anything and tried to educate me to tune into my body. She asked what symptoms I had been experiencing to which my only response was the pain in my wrist. She let me know that she found the effects in my hand, wrist, elbow, underarm, neck, cheek, eye and face on the left side of my body, the oesophagus, stomach, intestines, right groin and left kidney. She was very concerned about my left eye and left kidney, in particular. She suggested that Bowen therapy would also be beneficial. I left with an appointment to see her again in a week's time and an appointment for a Bowen therapy session with her husband, Paul.

Well, within the hour I had a massive headache. As soon as Mum looked at me she twigged. I had been suffering occasional headaches but we hadn't related it to the effects of the electrical burn. There hadn't been any specific pattern at this stage that we had observed. Mum mentioned this to me and also that this was what Judith was questioning me about in her consultation room.

This brought to mind the time physio Greg received a

really beaut zap from me that just about sent him through the wall — the crack was really loud. Being around computers had been causing a problem for me — I had a feeling of being spaced-out I suppose, sometimes headaches, and my left wrist pained enormously. The symptoms would somewhat dissipate once I was able to get away from the computer fields and into fresh air. I was beginning to realise that this zapping that was occurring fairly regularly and the effect of magnetic fields of electrical items were a consequence of the electrocution. I was to learn that even the electrical activity of an electrical storm would have an effect on me.

This headache was rather severe. Of course I swore at Mum for trying out her latest fangled idea of taking me to see Judith as my headaches hadn't been quite as bad as this one. Mum suggested some pain relief but I didn't want to take any as every time I had, since the accident, I ended up vomiting. I was also unsure if it would interfere with the healing session. I didn't want to do this without first checking with Judith. Mum said she was sure that it was the healing working unless I was reacting to the drops Judith had prescribed and she didn't see that some pain relief would create a problem. I took the drops and went off to bed without the pain relief and felt sick. The headache was unrelenting and I had it all night. Mum phoned Judith the next morning and asked if I could be reacting to the drops.

Judith was ecstatic to hear the effect the healing was having with me. She was very reassuring and explained what was occurring. She was even willing to fit me into her already full schedule for another session of healing earlier than the appointment allocated, to help relieve my pain if it was not subsiding over the next twenty-four hours. This says a lot about the type of person she is, as not many people are accommodating enough to even suggest this. It also affirmed her statement to me that she wasn't one for pain either, something that was important in my eyes. The next day, the severity of the headache lightened a little, although it was still with me and stayed with me for a few days. Mum and I decided to see how I travelled and to watch what was happening, so I kept my original appointment with Judith for the next week.

My second session of spiritual healing with Judith was on 26 March. Whilst at this session Judith was able to feel that the nerve was severed in my hand. She recommended a homoeopath to assist with my healing, as the two modalities combined are a hundred times more powerful than each on their own. This session of spiritual healing was immediately followed by Bowen therapy and an iridology session with Paul. I then continued on to school for the day and followed all instructions given.

When I returned home from school my brothers and sisters were looking at me weirdly. They wanted to know where all my energy had come from. They couldn't believe I was wanting to play ball with them. They kept asking Mum what had happened and if I was for real. You see, I had had no real energy since the accident back in July and when I came home from school I was normally so tired. It took all my energy to do my homework let alone play. My patience was always very low — the slightest thing would annoy me and I'd let everyone know. I had withdrawn a lot into myself since the accident, so the change in me was simply staggering to them all. I felt really good, full of life and, for a change, I was bounding with energy .

My second session of Bowen therapy with Paul was on 2 April. The homoeopath and the plastics specialist were consulted the following day. The homoeopath advised that we were looking at healing over a long term, probably around six months for the type of injury I had sustained.

We went on to see the plastics specialist, who immediately detected that my left arm was notably thinner than my right arm. He ordered a bone-density scan of my left hand and wrist. We asked if he had any problems with alternative healing modalities and spoke to him of Judith and what she had discovered. His first question was, 'What are her credentials?'. The doctor took a copy of the flier I had, and said I could keep going with it as long as it worked. Neither Mum nor I mentioned the rest of what we had been doing apart from seeing Judith. I was determined to keep travelling with these alternative methods of healing no matter what, as they were accomplishing far more than what had been offered to me through traditional medicine and to date that was very little.

During this period I saw Judith for a further seven sessions of spiritual healing. In these sessions it was like peeling away the layers of an onion. Layer after layer, more and more was revealed each time. The shoulder was a big block. This was mentioned to the homoeopath and the drops prescribed helped break up this area. The effect of the electricity was found in my nerves, muscle, bone and even the blood. It was found in the left eye socket, behind the eye, the cheek bone, the nasal area, the left lung. The effects were staggering. I learnt to become more in tune with my body and to identify exactly where the pain or symptom was occurring: for example, when I was experiencing a headache, whether it was at the front of my head or towards the back. There is a difference and it is of significance. At one stage I was experiencing two headaches together and I could tell you exactly where they were. I had learnt and am still learning to tune in to my body.

Whenever I saw the homoeopath, I would tell him what was happening in spiritual healing and when I next saw Judith, I would tell her what the homoeopath had said and prescribed. I only needed to see the homoeopath for a total of three sessions because the healing came much faster than anticipated. I also let Judith know what was happening with the specialist.

During the period I was seeing Judith I ceased my visits to the physiotherapist. The day I last saw Judith was also the day I saw the specialist, and just a few days short of being twelve months from the date of the accident. He informed me that he knew I would always get better and get back the use of my hand. He said that I had more chance of regaining the function of my hand than either he or Mum in the same situation, as youth was on my side. Mum didn't agree with this comment.

I don't see how I would have obtained my healing if I had stayed solely with traditional medicine, considering that my recovery had plateaued under it and that they could not do anything more. Monitoring appears to be all they could offer me.

At present I have discovered that I can rub a spot in my wrist and I can feel a sensation in the back of my hand, and if I touch a certain spot in my elbow I can feel it in my hand. This sensation is my latest toy to play with.

I have improved immensely since first seeing Judith. I know that quite a substantial amount of my healing took place through her giftedness. Even my mates at school have commented on the strength that has returned, especially to my left side.

I believe, most firmly, that the recovery of the initial function to my hand was with the help, encouragement and perseverance of physio Greg. Furthermore, if I hadn't sought alternative healing, and come upon the richness of Judith's healing gift, I possibly would not be where I am today — a glowing picture of health and vitality. I am walking proof of her abilities.

Carmel's story — Brain tumour

On Sunday, 17 April 1994, I awoke with the right side of my face paralysed. My first thoughts were that I had had a stroke, but on realising that I could move my body I was relieved that this was not the case. This did not lessen my terror about my face. I had no idea what was wrong with me.

A visit to my family friend and GP confirmed that I had Bell's palsy. (I had never heard of this.) To be on the safe side my doctor referred me for a CAT scan.

The scan was done the next day with the result showing a growth in the mastoid. After being referred to a specialist I was told that the tumour had eroded the seventh nerve in the face and that a major reconstruction of this nerve would be needed if I was to get any movement back in my face. I was to be admitted to the RPA the next Wednesday for surgery the following day.

On my return from the specialist, I called Judith whom I had consulted on a previous occasion. I told her of my problem and asked her to pray for me. She replied that she would do more than that and I should visit her the following Tuesday. My daughter drove me to see Judith for the healing session, which lasted about twenty minutes. She said not to worry, that they would decide not to operate and that the condition would not be what it appeared to be.

At the RPA on the Wednesday a group of visiting specialists wanted to see me. They were confused as to why I had never had any pain or symptoms. My doctor noticed a slight flicker in my eye which was not there the previous week. After further consultation it was decided that the operation would not be carried out on the Thursday but they would wait one week to see if and how much my face improved.

During that week I had several sessions with Judith, and with each session my family could see improvement with my face. On entering the hospital the next week my doctor was shocked at how much my face had improved. The words he used were 'amazing' and 'extraordinary'. He had never seen such an improvement in such a short period of time. He thought this meant that the original prognosis with regard to the seventh nerve was wrong and that the tumour had not damaged it. It was decided, however, that the tumour operation would still go ahead.

The operation took place a few days later. On awaking from surgery I was told that there was 'no tumour' and that they could only conclude that my problem had been a herniated brain.

I continued to visit Judith to help with my recovery after the operation. Through the whole ordeal she helped me to retain a positive attitude. After each visit I felt better and within a few months I was back at work and very grateful that I had been spared.

I feel Judith can help people with problems such as mine. I cannot explain my wonderful results. I can only say that I believe Judith has spiritual healing power and is able to help people in desperate situations.

Victoria's story — Consistent migraine

I had suffered at least one migraine a month for the last eighteen months. I had been on medication three times a day or more when attacks hit.

I first heard of Judith Collins through an advertisement in the local paper. I attended an evening session with her which was informative but not for me at the time.

In March 1997, after being sick of seeing a chiropractor every month for my back and neck pain, I visited Paul Collins (Judith's husband) for Bowen therapy. While under treatment I suffered one of my 'migraines' and was advised to see Judith.

After two visits to Judith I felt a vast improvement: the number of attacks had fallen and medication had been reduced.

I am still seeing Judith. I am looking forward to further improvements and discovering myself.

Valerie's story — Persistent migraine

For nearly seven years I had suffered extremely debilitating headaches. I had gone from one doctor to another in search of someone who would diagnose and 'fix' whatever was causing me to suffer with these 'blinders' everyday for all those years. I was referred to many 'specialist' doctors ranging from a neurologist who prescribed tablets with so many side-effects that the 'cure' was worse than the complaint, to a 'specialist' ENT man who said my 'bite' was maligned. Needless to say, none of these so-called experts were able to pinpoint or cure my headaches (one doctor even hinted that I was imagining it all!). I endured all sorts of analyses such as blood tests for thyroid function, CAT scans for brain tumours, metal probes inserted into each nostril to 'check' my sinuses — most uncomfortable to say the least!!

For about sixteen months my sister and a work colleague had been trying to persuade me to go and see Judith Collins but my reply was 'I don't believe in mumbo-jumbo and I doubt anything can be done'. However, after a particularly bad four days where I was barely able to function at work and despite my usual 12–15 tablets per day, I decided that maybe a little mumbo-jumbo just might fix my problem. I was truly desperate and willing to be subjected to anything. The very next day I rang for an appointment with Judith and was told that due to a cancellation I would be able to see her the next morning. The rest, as they say, is history!

After only a few moments with Judith she was able to tell me that my headaches were being caused by problems within my pituitary gland but this did not pose a major drama and that she would simply 'heal' me, which she did in a matter of minutes. During the healing I had a feeling of extreme calm and warmth throughout my body. Judith explained that this was my body healing itself and suggested whenever I experienced this to just give in and allow the healing to progress. I had one more visit with Judith and she was not surprised when I told her I had not had one headache in a whole week. I was and still am absolutely amazed. I have been almost headache-free since then. Occasionally I may experience a 'bad-head-day' but the pain does not last and is usually due to a hectic nine- or ten-hour day at work! I am no longer a shareholder with the drug companies.

Thank-you Judith Collins. You are one warm, beautiful lady who will forever have my admiration and thanks.

Gertrude's story — Long term injury

In 1979 I had a car accident and damaged an upper conic disc in the lower back. In addition I suffered severe whiplash so my whole spine was very painful. This condition persisted for twelve years without respite. During this period the doctor who treated me prescribed pain-killer drugs. I also received physiotherapy.

Approximately four years ago I heard about Judith Collins through a Radio 2UE programme, which provided details of a healing circle to be held at Penrith. During the circle Judith put her hands on my shoulders and I felt a warm healing sensation. That evening I made an appointment to see her at Earthkeepers.

At the consultation I lay down on a table, Judith put her hands on my body and I could feel healing forces taking place. Over a period of four weeks my condition improved considerably.

I had had an operation on my left big toe which had resulted in the toe being rigid. I had been unable to bend this toe for fifty years. I was pleasantly surprised that as a result of Judith's treatment I can now bend this toe to an extent not experienced since the operation.

Louise's story — Chronic fatigue

Over a period of two years I suffered from chronic fatigue syndrome and experienced constant pressure in my head, and headaches that lasted up to three weeks at a time. My eyesight was affected. I had 'tunnel vision', sensitivity to light and eye pain. I had constant sinusitis. My joints ached. My body ached. I had diarrhoea. I lost weight. I suffered fevers and tingling sensations in my hands and feet that were so severe it was painful. My hearing was affected and I lost my sense of smell. I had a continuous post-nasal drip that was affecting my taste. I experienced extreme tiredness. It felt like massive exhaustion all the time. I slept at least twelve hours a night and two to three hours every afternoon. I suffered short term memory loss and an inability to concentrate. I also contracted glandular fever and pneumonia. I simply did not get better.

I had seen four doctors (GPs), a lung specialist (for the pneumonia), and an ENT specialist who did two operations.

There was little improvement. Since the doctors could not find out why I was not getting better, the ENT specialist did a tonsillectomy (it was thought that my tonsils might be poisoning my system). I also had a nose operation (to clear out the nose and sinus).

I went to an eye specialist who could find nothing wrong except fatigue. I had a CAT scan and they could not find anything wrong except inflammation of the sinus near the base of the brain. I went to a dentist and had metal fillings removed for fear of mercury poisoning but that didn't help. I saw a naturopath who tried Reiki healing and counselling. I went to a herbalist who gave me tonics. I also had an aromatherapy massage.

The medical profession were at a loss as to how to further treat me. Months of antibiotics had left my immune system completely run down. I was frustrated and scared. The medical profession said they did not know what to do. I cried. I stayed suspended in a state of debilitating illness and extreme fatigue. My life was a living nightmare. It had come to a standstill.

After about twelve months, my energy slowly increased, inch by inch, a little each month but the progress was excruciatingly slow. With the smallest amount of over-exertion I would regress to a state of acute illness and fatigue that would take weeks to recover from. The medical profession had abandoned me. I was dealing with my condition on my own.

Out of the blue I enrolled in an Aura Energy course held once a fortnight for six sessions. I had not attended anything like this before. It opened my eyes and heart to natural therapies and healing. I was then drawn extraordinarily to the book *How to See and Read the Human Aura* by Judith Collins. It just seemed to jump out at me in a bookshop. After reading this book I knew that I would seek out Judith Collins and that she would be able to help me.

I remember the first time I met Judith she was shining. I could hardly see where I was going yet I felt her warmth and energy. I felt like I was in the presence of an angel. The only effort I had to make was to relax. There was no counselling, lecturing nor even too much talking which was a great relief as I had difficulty listening, speaking or even following directions. I did not know what was wrong with me, so it was a great relief to find that Judith did not expect me to know either. But Judith knew. I could tell she knew and I accepted where I was at. So she knew where to start to heal. She knew just by looking at me.

The treatment took only about ten minutes. I just relaxed while Judith healed my body with the touch of her hands. Judith diagnosed two glands that had a major malfunction: the thymus and the pituitary.

For the next four days I felt as though I had just stepped out of soaking in a lovely warm bath. My body was at ease for the first time in two years.

I visited Judith Collins at Earthkeepers about once a month for the next six months. It was my life line, my last resort, my only hope. At first my progress was slow and steady but was always with ease. My energy was returning. Then my headaches disappeared. During the last two months my progress was so rapid. I could see clearly again! I was smiling and laughing. I was almost in a state of disbelief. All pain had left my body.

The wonderful thing about Judith's healing is that there is no pain, no side-effects and no trauma. The other amazing thing is that some other pre-existing symptoms disappeared as well. I no longer suffer from heavy PMT. My lower back ache has also disappeared.

When everything else had failed, when all else had given up on me, Judith was there. I only wish I had discovered Judith's healing powers sooner. Earthkeepers was my last hope for complete recovery before I gave up my life.

For me, chronic fatigue syndrome was a most debilitating illness. It filled me with frustration and despair, plunging me into the darkest hours of my life. Judith Collins' healing gave me back my quality of life. It is my hope that other people will find their way to Judith to be restored to good health as I was. Do not be afraid to be healed in this gentle and effective way.

Thank-you Judith with all my heart.

Lyn's story — Life-restricting migraine

I have suffered from migraines for twenty years. In that time I have had teeth pulled out and acupuncture. I have seen an osteopath (which did help a little bit) and have been on a course of preventative pills.

A friend of mine recommended Bowen therapy with Paul Collins, which in turn led to a consultation with Judith.

The results have been astounding. From suffering two or three times a day, it is now down to two or three times a month. I have a whole new life. The migraines are now not so severe. Also I am taking less pills than before.

Judith Collins has helped me a great deal more than any other type of treatment.

Lila's story — Emotional damage and childhood trauma

I met Judith four or five years ago at Earthkeepers Healing Sanctuary. I felt Judith could answer my questions and would be able to help me.

I had not been well for a long time, both physically and emotionally. In general I had not been happy. There were a lot of issues regarding my childhood and family that I had been carrying around with me. At the time she told me a lot of things about myself which she could not have known unless you knew me well, but we had just met.

She made me realise my strengths and weaknesses and see what I was really like. We discussed my parents and family. I don't think I understood the meaning of everything she said then, but she put my mind at ease. I felt this connection with her at my first appointment and I felt a sense of calmness and love.

Soon after I began visits to Judith, my husband started to see changes in me. I was happy and had a very positive attitude towards life.

I was brought up as a Catholic and as a kid loved churches and religion, but growing up I could not identify with God. Since I have met Judith I feel that no matter what happens, there is always a way out and there is a reason for being in this realm of life.

Healing was an appropriate step for me to take at the time. It was a tremendous experience. During sessions with Judith my whole body felt wonderful. I would feel this warmth travelling through my arms and hands. I hated the end of the sessions because you just wanted to continue with the same wonderful state of mind and body.

Judith has touched my soul in a manner that has allowed me to grow and see life from a totally different perspective, allowing me to see what I need and am looking for. The effect has been so profound that it has affected not just myself but my family as well. We were able to find the right help when one of my children was unwell.

Whenever I listen to a friend, hear the radio or watch television, there is all this information that I can now absorb. I could not do this before.

All the worries in my world appear not to be worries any longer. I just face life and make the most of it and ask God to give me the strength to learn with dignity.

Fay's story — Smoker's congested lungs

For many years I had suffered from bronchitis, sometimes for weeks at a time. The treatment I was receiving from the doctors meant taking prescription drugs, sometimes with undesirable side effects.

I got to know about Judith when my sister and I went to a natural health show at Camden, after reading an advertisement in a newspaper. During the day I was handed a brochure about Earthkeepers Healing Sanctuary, which I put on file. One day, by chance, I came across the brochure. I was so pleased I had kept it.

I had caught the flu and this was followed by bronchitis. The antibiotics were helping very little as my lungs were holding so much fluid. I was feeling poorly. I decided to go and see Judith at Earthkeepers for help. After the first visit I felt improvement. Judith was able to clear all the congestion from my lungs despite the fact that I was smoking at the time.

Jan's story — Throat and breathing condition

I am a fifty-two year old mother of three. I was born in NSW and moved to Victoria in 1961 when my father was transferred on business.

I experienced a bout of illness at six years of age when I developed whooping cough, mumps and pneumonia that resulted in my absence from school for six months. I was always an active or, as my parents would say, 'overactive' child. I didn't like to walk anywhere; I was always running. The only time my running slowed me down was after a recurrent bout of pneumonia at eleven years of age. I found that whenever I ran for long periods of time, for example, during hockey matches at school, which I loved, it took two hours for me to stop wheezing. By the time my parents arrived home I had recovered; they didn't realise I had a breathing problem at this stage.

I took up swimming training at twelve years of age after meeting the Australian swimming team whilst on holidays in Townsville with my family. The team was preparing for the 1956 Olympics. I was most impressed, and it was at this stage that I decided that one day I wanted to represent Australia at the Olympics as well. With a lot of dedicated work from my parents, my coaches and myself I achieved my dream of being chosen as a member of the 1964 Olympic swimming team.

Over the years I had always had a weak chest however my swimming career most certainly helped me by strengthening my lungs and keeping me fitter than I otherwise would have been.

After my swimming career ended, I gradually developed a weakness in my lungs, which was much more noticeable after a bout of Bell's palsy and glandular fever in 1989. I spent eight months recovering to a stage where I could re-enter the workforce and resume my career on a part-time basis as a consultant with Drake International. I was still very drained and experiencing headaches, a slight cough and a very sore right side of my head. The medical profession had assured me that I was going through post-viral syndrome and that the symptoms would gradually disappear. I returned to full-time employment after ten months. In the early stages of my recovery I had regular chiropractic treatment which helped my headaches and gradually I began to feel stronger.

Five years ago I joined the Major Engineering Group as their Human Resources Manager which I find a very challenging and rewarding position. About four years ago my chest condition worsened. At this stage I was having antibiotics and various sprays for the continuing coughing and lung infections. I had numerous tests for allergies and asthma. After taking the antibiotics the symptoms would cease for a period of a month or so, and then would reoccur.

Approximately two years ago I was diagnosed with chronic bronchitis, which included coughing continually, especially at night. Then I experienced regular nose bleeds and was not able to walk 400 metres without gasping for breath.

At this time I decided I had experienced enough of traditional medical treatment and that I wanted to try other avenues. I went to my first *Mind, Body and Spirit Festival* where I sourced various modalities that I felt may help me get to the cause of the problem rather than continuing with the band-aid procedures I had experienced so far. These included kinesiology, homoeopathy, massage and Chinese herbalism. I had improved somewhat and they had all played a part in the healing process; however, I knew I needed something else.

I had seen Judith Collins at the *Mind, Body and Spirit Festival* and I was intrigued by what I had seen, read and heard in relation to her healing abilities. I had previously attended an aura reading/training session with her. Then I received some information from the Earthkeepers Healing Sanctuary in relation to the *Festival of Health and Harmony* and discovered that Judith would be holding private healing consultations whilst in Melbourne where I made an appointment to see her in October 1997.

Judith informed me of my childhood chest problems and also remarked that I had a sore ear (Bell's palsy) without my mentioning either of these. This certainly made me feel at ease and I was amazed at her perception and knowledge of these ailments. I felt confident that Judith would be able to help me.

During my healing session with Judith I experienced extreme heat in my chest and on my head. The heat reoccurred in my chest whilst driving home and at various times throughout the next few days, along with other symptoms I was advised may occur. These included rumbling noises in my abdomen, specific heat surges, pains in my head and sinuses, aching in my right ear and tingling in my arms and hands. After the first few days I felt a lightness in my whole body as though I was floating along — I felt taller.

Because of my swimming background I am quite in tune with subtle changes that occur within my body and so I found this an extremely interesting experience. I actually had two nights where I slept without coughing; I could not believe it. I was so excited when I went to see Judith for my next appointment that I could not keep quiet.

Three weeks later I am much improved and continuing with the consultations. Hopefully I will be able to have my condition under control or be fully recovered in the next three months. I realise that to have a complete recovery my body needs to be balanced emotionally, physically, structurally and spiritually. After the last eight years of being unwell, and searching intuitively for answers I needed to know, I have experienced personal growth and encountered many interesting and enlightened people. I feel positive and feel that this stage of my life is a great opportunity for me to clear any negativity. I look forward to an exciting and healthy future with my family and friends and in professional life.

Maureen's story — Arthritis

In mid-1995 I developed arthritis in both knees, which resulted in constant pain. I tried all the accepted treatments including anti-flammatory tablets, creams and gels that I applied externally to both knees, acupuncture, dietary changes and natural remedies. None of these things worked.

After fourteen months of continuous pain I attended one of Judith Collins' healing circles. While taking part in the circle I was surprised to find that the pain in my knees subsided. I was so impressed that I went to see Judith for a private consultation and after three consecutive healing sessions the arthritic pain in my knees went away completely.

I am thoroughly convinced that without Judith's intervention I would still be experiencing this painful condition.

Alec's story — Reduced medication for diabetes

Before I had a healing from Judith I was on insulin and four diamicron per day to control my diabetes. My blood–sugar readings were around twenty prior to using insulin.

Since the healing I have not taken insulin (apart from a period when I had pleurisy) but have remained on tablets, and my blood–sugar readings have dropped to six.

I continue with the healings three or four times per year as they contribute greatly to my general well-being. I feel the healing go right through my body.

Thank-you Judith.

Sharon's story — Painful menstruation

I came to work at Earthkeepers Healing Sanctuary as Judith Collins' secretary in February 1997. I will always remember my first day working there because I was not feeling the best.

I was coming up to my menstrual cycle and it was having a bit of trouble starting. I have always suffered from stomach cramps prior to menstruating and this particular day was worse than ever before. The pain was excruciating.

I was suffering from sharp pains in my stomach and a feeling of nausea. I was doubled over in pain when Judith came in to see me. She immediately got me up on the massage table and put her hands on the side of my stomach. I did not mention what was wrong with me but just let her know that my stomach was hurting.

I could feel the heat generating from Judith's hands and it was very soothing. Judith told me that there was nothing to worry about, that it was just my menstrual cycle, and that the egg was trying to pull away and was having difficulty in doing so. She told me that I could feel a pulling sensation in my stomach and I was amazed because that was exactly what I could feel.

After a short time she asked me how I felt and upon standing I was surprised to feel no pain at all. I felt fine for the rest of the day and my period began straight afterwards. For many months following this I had pain-free periods.

I have seen many sick people come to see Judith and it makes me feel proud to work for her as she helps so many people. People come in looking sick and after seeing Judith for a consultation they come out looking so much better. It always makes me feel good to see the relief in their eyes after Judith has eased some of their pain.

The only drawback in working for a spiritual healer is that I can never ring up and say I need to have a day off, using the excuse that I am sick, because Judith will just tell me to come in and she will do her healing on me!

People often ask me if the healing really works and I can honestly tell them it does. I have felt it myself and have seen with my own eyes that it works on other people.

Thank-you Judith for all the help that you have given me and everyone else. I feel very honoured to work for you.

Caroline's story — Breast cancer

I was diagnosed with breast cancer in December 1996. I underwent two operations, in December 1996 and February 1997, and commenced a course of chemotherapy in March. It was at this time that a friend suggested I make an appointment to see Judith — she had been to see her and spoke highly of her.

Early breast cancer is an insidious disease. It lies in wait, poised to strike again when you think you have overcome it. There may be no physical signs of its presence until a routine check discovers it has spread and is on a death march inside your body.

So a diagnosis of breast cancer forced me to face many issues such as the fear of pain and the possibility of death, but perhaps the hardest was the uncertainty. It is said that the possibility of dying of cancer exists until you die of something else! Having said that, cancer does also give you an opportunity and indeed a compelling reason to change your life. For someone like me, perhaps more importantly, it gave permission to change.

At the time I first saw Judith I was coping reasonably well with the aftermath of the operations and the effects of chemotherapy. After seeing her, I felt a change, in that I was no longer trying to cope, I was simply healing.

Seeing Judith has helped me in many ways. I am sure she helped to improve my mental state — for several days after first seeing her, in a floaty sort of way I was on a natural 'high'. Following that, I felt at peace and more in touch and in tune with myself, my body and the world around me. Kind of like being 'in the flow' of life. This in itself made it much easier for me to cope with all the extra stresses caused by my illness and to take steps to improve my life in various ways. What it has meant for me is peace of mind, acceptance, increased awareness, appreciation ... I really can't explain or quantify it, but I simply felt better!

Another thing I have really appreciated about Judith is her wisdom — sometimes I can't see the woods for the trees. She has helped me to see things in a different way and to clarify many things in my mind with her wise and simple suggestions and answers. I do believe Judith helped me to be a better person, even though this is an ongoing and arduous task!

Apart from that, Judith displays a wicked sense of humour on occasion, and her workshops are fun and illuminating as well as inspiring. Likewise are her tapes and her books, which I have read and re-read.

I admire and appreciate Judith for many things.

Laurie's story — Angina

My story starts in mid-1989, at 55 years of age, when my wife for 29 years plus (who was experiencing menopause) informed me that she wished to sell our lovely home, take half each and go our separate ways. At first I did not take her seriously, but she soon made me realise that she was serious. Despite my efforts to resolve the situation it was obvious her mind was made up.

We put the house up for auction but it failed to meet our reserve price. Then began a long process of 'open days' for public inspection in order to dispose of the family home. I found this very distressing, as well as the fact that my wife was gradually withdrawing from me. She had moved into the spare room months earlier and was making a point of not talking to me. At this stage I must mention that I was, and still am, a staunch believer in the family unit. Up to that time, I was very proud of the way we operated as a family. We had been blessed with two lovely children: the eldest a son who, at the time, was 27 years of age and a daughter who was 25 years of age. No parent could have wished for better children. I felt totally shattered that my family unit was breaking down. I was losing my wife, my house and my self-respect. My world was falling apart around me and I could do nothing to stop it.

Christmas 1989 was very strained. I remember thinking that I would not see another Christmas in that beautiful home. The New Year passed and 1990 started very poorly. I was most unhappy and kept thinking that somehow something would happen to make things better.

On 31 January 1990 I woke up, had breakfast and left for work at 7:30 am. I was about 1.5 kilometres down the road when I started to sweat profusely. The morning was rather cool and I could not understand why I was suddenly sweating. I was feeling terrible but I had been feeling that way for months. I then felt this sharp, deep penetrating pain in the centre of my chest, I knew then I was in trouble. I told myself to stay calm and think. I was in peak hour traffic. I knew I had to get to hospital. If I stopped to get help or get a lift, people would think I was drunk or on drugs. I decided I would drive myself to hospital which was about 10 kilometres away. I was on the main road and it was a fairly direct run.

The next 20 minutes felt like an eternity. The pain spread across my chest and into the tops of my arms. My face, head and body were saturated with sweat but I was able to stay calm because I had somebody talking to me, telling me I would make it, that I would be alright and not to worry. At no time did I feel afraid. The pain was excruciating but I kept saying to myself 'It's only pain — it won't kill you'. Nearing the hospital I had to make a sharp left hand turn, and even now I can clearly recall yelling out with the pain in my arms as I pulled the steering wheel around. I kept thinking maybe this is some sort of nightmare.

On arriving at the hospital my next concern was, can I make it to the Emergency counter? I got out of the car and steadied myself against the side of the vehicle. I then said to myself: 'You've made it this far. Don't mess it up now'. I slowly but surely walked into the reception foyer and across to the counter but there was nobody there. I was holding tightly onto the counter and I heard a voice ask 'May I help you?'. As I turned towards her I said 'I have severe chest pain'. She took one look at me and ran off and arrived back with a wheelchair. Within minutes I was on a bed in Emergency, stripped off and having monitor leads fixed to my chest. I was still sweating profusely and even after two anguine tablets, I was still in a lot of pain. After two hours in Emergency they told me I was to be admitted, and that I would now be taken to the Coronary Care Unit. On arrival there, the sister met me at the bed and told the orderlies to put me on the bed. She stripped the gown from me and started swabbing me with cold towels, which I must say felt wonderful. She soon settled me down and poured me a glass of water which, to my amazement, I could not pick up. She quickly assured me that it often happens that one suffers complete exhaustion after experiencing a coronary attack.

The following morning the doctor and coronary sisters called on me during their rounds. The doctor stated that it had been confirmed that I had suffered a heart attack.

I immediately replied that they were wrong and that there must be some mistake. I did not want to accept that my body had failed me. In my mind, only old and frail people suffered heart attacks. I was too young, too fit, too strong.

In hindsight, my thinking was that I did not want to suffer another loss. What with my marriage, my home and my family unit, another failure was something I could not accept. I felt that I was in a nose dive. I was going down and there was no way I could stop it. Despair and depression were weighing heavily on me.

I arrived home ten days later a very weak, frightened and confused person, the slightest twinge in my body terrified me. I began attending rehabilitation courses which were very beneficial to my recovery and I resumed work the beginning of May 1990, exactly twelve weeks after suffering the attack.

1990 was a year of fluctuating emotions, temperament and security. My wife was intolerant with my ill health and my inability to work around the home. In late 1990 I went to see a psychologist named Jim. It was due to Jim that I was able to begin getting my life in order. It was not long after this time that my wife moved out of the family home. I was not upset, as our relationship had become impossible. Jim changed my whole attitude towards myself and my perception of life.

I had been of the belief that life was a competition where your worth was measured by the number of victories you had, that we had to be better than our fellow man, and that any form of failure was unacceptable whereby you were looked down on by your peers. I had to live my life to the expectations others placed on me. I had to be whoever or whatever others wanted me to be. I had to be liked and accepted by everybody. I believed I was the number one 'macho man'.

Jim changed all of that. He made me throw away the masks, get rid of the camouflage and accept myself for who I am and what I am. He made me realise how much life has to offer by keeping our lives on a simple plane. By only allowing ourselves to be excited and overjoyed by the unusual and spectacular, we rob ourselves of the joys, pleasures and excitement of everyday life. We live in our own worlds through the places we frequent with people who come in and out of our lives and our friends and families. If we treat each other with love, respect and caring we can create a beautiful warm glow within our world, where we each develop a feeling of dignity and healthy self-esteem, and where stress and anger drain from our beings and are replaced by peace and freedom. That is the ideal we should all be aiming for.

In late 1990 our daughter informed us that she was expecting a baby. This news was a ray of light, providing me with great pleasure in what had been a disastrous year. I was looking towards 1991 with great anticipation.

In February my son asked me if I would move in with him for the month of April. As my wife was due to have a hysterectomy and as his home had stairs in the front and rear, it would be easier for her if she moved into the family home. I agreed that it would be easier for her in the family home but I could not see the reason for me to move out. A very heated argument took place and he left the house in a raging temper. I was totally distraught by the experience.

In March my first grandchild, Lisa-Maree, was born twenty weeks premature and died twenty minutes after birth. My daughter and son-in-law were heartbroken and both sides of the family were devastated as Lisa-Maree would have been the first grandchild for both grandparents.

In April my father-in-law died of a heart attack after complications. I was very deeply saddened by his passing. For many years we worked together in partnership as builders. He was my mate, my friend, and was a warm, generous person.

In late April my mother had several strokes and was admitted to hospital in a coma. I can clearly recall sitting by her bed, holding her hand and saying: 'How can you leave me now? I've lost everything and now you are going. Please stay a while longer'.

In early May the funeral for Lisa-Maree took place in the hospital chapel. Once again it was a time of great sadness. What could have been a wonderful and exciting time in our lives had been taken from us.

In mid-May my mother passed away after being in a coma for several weeks. I was completely shattered. My wife kept visiting me in the family home, wanting to know why it hadn't yet been sold. Eventually she rang the agent and accepted a price we had previously regarded as being too low. It was arranged that I move out of the family home in November.

In September, after weeks of flat-hunting, I bought a beautiful unit in a court setting. I now reside there very happily.

In January 1992 I noticed that I was experiencing more chest pain. As I knew I could relieve it with anguine tablets, I was not greatly concerned. By 31 January I was once again admitted to hospital. I received angioplasty treatment on 10 February 1992 and have enjoyed freedom from chest pain since then.

In June 1992 I suffered an attack of deep depression and decided to visit my psychologist friend Jim again. In total we had ten sessions and they all involved 'grieving'. He said so much had happened in such a short time that I had been unable to deal with it, so I had suppressed my feelings. During the treatment period I cried continuously for three weeks. I would be driving in my car and for no apparent reason I would burst into tears. I could be watching television and the same thing would happen. He explained that I would continue to have fits of depression but they would not be as deep and that they would be less frequent.

In July 1997 my daughter arranged a healing appointment for me during Judith Collins' stay in Melbourne. After the consultation I felt great inner peace and calmed right down. I was quick to notice that my anxiety attacks had been healed. The healing was wonderful.

In October that year, following my periodic medical examination, I was told that my blood test and ECG showed I was completely free of both the symptoms and angina.

In looking back over those years I believe that in spite of the times of anguish and heartbreak, I am a better person for having been through it. My values and priorities have changed, my attitudes have changed and I aspire to life from a more positive and optimistic perspective.

To me life is challenging, exciting and wonderful. I acknowledge and appreciate my world, my family and friends and this wonderful life God has given me.

Noel's story — Emphysema

About four years ago I was suffering from pains in my chest and could not breathe properly. I went to the hospital for a check-up and they diagnosed me with emphysema.

Soon after, I attended the *Mind, Body and Spirit Festival* in

Sydney and it was there that I picked up some brochures on Judith Collins. I was then sent some more brochures from my wife's friend who told me that Judith was soon going to be in Newcastle to conduct a healing circle.

I attended the healing circle and the next day my coughing had ceased. It felt as though everything in my chest had moved and I was bringing up a lot of phlegm. I felt really good. I then booked several appointments with Judith at her clinic at Earthkeepers.

Since returning to doctors they have made comments on how well I am now. My wife is also pleased with the results. Before I saw Judith, I was always up all night coughing and my wife could not sleep properly. Now the coughing has calmed down and we are both able to sleep. I used to get panic attacks before as well but now I don't experience these either.

I speak highly of Judith. She has put years onto my life. I have had friends die from emphysema because they were not fortunate enough to have met Judith. I am grateful for the help that Judith has given me.

Betty's story — Thrombosis

I had a healing consultation with Judith in October 1997 after I'd had a series of falls and my knees especially were damaged.

I limped into her Melbourne clinic and walked out normally. When Judith placed her healing hands on my knees, the right knee became burning hot and the left knee became icy cold. For good measure she attended to my thrombosed legs which have bothered me for the last thirty years.

Since Christmas 1997 I have resumed my morning walks — slowly at first but now a kilometre in fifteen minutes. I no longer suffer from tired, aching legs. I might add that I am sixty-eight years old and am more fit now than I was thirty years ago.

Judith, you have given me a second chance through your wonderful healing hands for which I am eternally grateful.

Wilma's story — Whiplash

Out of curiosity I attended Judith's healing circle at the *Conscious Living Expo* in Perth in 1996.

I advised Judith of a sight condition only. I did not mention neck injuries from three motor vehicle accidents over a period of eight years.

The spike on which the head rotates was out of alignment, causing a lot of pain and often severe headaches. There was also tenderness at the base of the skull and in parts of the scalp.

It was about a week after the workshop that I suddenly realised I'd had no pain since attending the healing circle. One month later I no longer had pain at the base of my skull and I had much greater rotation of my neck. Once I had been told that it was incurable!

The fee for the workshop was well worth the benefits I am reaping now. I am doing things that I haven't done for years! 'Thank-you' seems so little to say for the improved quality of life you have given me.

6 AFFIRMING GOOD HEALTH AND RECOVERY

THE ROAD to good health and recovery can be helped by positive assertion in all areas of your life. Developing and utilising the power of positive thinking can assist in reprogramming the mind for the reduction and/or the release of illness. Follow this fourteen-day active affirmation programme and notice the subtle changes in your intention, thoughts and well-being.

To create the appropriate environment for affirming good health and recovery, each morning on waking, take seven deep and gentle breaths. Close your eyes and use your mind to examine your body for imbalance, discomfort and disease. Start at the feet and work up to the top of the head. On completion, say the affirmation aloud several times, working the voice from its usual pitch and volume level, to a faint whisper. Repeat once silently.

I suggest that you lie with your feet slightly raised on a pillow, or sit in a comfortable chair with your back straight and with your feet evenly spaced and planted firmly on the ground. Your hands should be facing upwards to encourage the flow of the body's energy.

As inspiration and self-questioning arises, don't hesitate or procrastinate in searching for answers and resources. It's handy to have a small notepad next to you so that as thoughts and issues arise with the challenge of the affirmation you can jot them down when the affirmation process is complete.

The thought for the day acts as a trigger to assist the affirmation process and should therefore be the focus of your thinking at every available moment throughout the day. Should you gain some insight or find that questions arise, be sure to make a note of them for further self-examination, so that this major part of the self-healing process may be thoroughly addressed.

The last seven days of the affirmations can be repeated until you reach your desired goal.

The fourteen-day programme of affirmations begins on page 119.

How to Activate Self-Healing

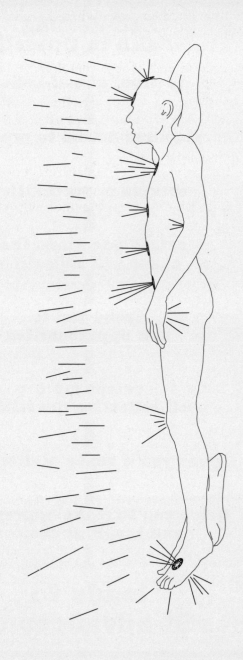

To activate self-healing, lie down with your head supported by a pillow. Place your hands on the crest of the groin. Take seven deep breaths through the nostrils, and exhale very slowly through the mouth. Repeat the self-healing invocation on page 57.

Self-Healing
Faith in Oneself

is proof of self-belief

requires action to prove it

creates opportunities

raises questions that
cause self-reflection

opens you to
new opportunities

raises more
self-reflective questions

gives you a sense of direction

helps you to make appropriate
and inspired choices

leads to
self-advancement

Developing
the Self-Healing
Disposition

1
Find joy in relationships

2
Find contentment
in daily routines

3
Find love
in
self-reflection

4
Find peace in recreation

5
Find hope in thoughts

6
Find life in everything

Living in Peace

*
Never debate, discuss

*
Never threaten
a person's beliefs
as everyone has their own truth

*
Look for the goodness
in everyone

*
Establish a common ground
with others' beliefs
so that acceptance flows

*
Know that
your path of self-healing
is reflective,
Others may learn
by your example

*
Give service without question

DAY 1

Thought for the Day
I AM POWERFUL

Affirmation

I have the power within to facilitate my own healing.
My intention is clear. I plan to overcome this affliction.
I honour my affliction for what it is teaching me about myself.
I look for the lessons it offers.

DAY 2

Thought for the Day
I CARE

Affirmation

I honour my affliction for what it is teaching me.
I look for the lessons it offers.
I challenge myself to resolve it.

DAY 3

Thought for the Day
I SEEK

Affirmation

I honour my affliction for what it is teaching me.
I look for the lessons it offers.
I search for the direction of healing.

DAY 4

Thought for the Day
A NEW BEGINNING

Affirmation

I honour my affliction for what it is teaching me.
I look for the lessons it offers.
I am the direction of healing.
The healing begins within me.

DAY 5

Thought for the Day
 SELF-VALUE

Affirmation

I honour my affliction for what it is teaching me.
I look for the lessons it offers.
Through self-recognition the healing has begun.

DAY 6

Thought for the Day
SELF-UNDERSTANDING

Affirmation

I honour my affliction for what it is teaching me.
I look for the lessons it offers.
Through self-understanding the healing has begun.

DAY 7

Thought for the Day
THE POWER OF THE MIND

Affirmation

I honour my affliction for what it is teaching me.
I look for the lessons it offers.
Through the power of my mind the healing has begun.

DAY 8

Thought for the Day
SELF-ANALYSIS

Affirmation

I honour my affliction for what it is teaching me.
I look for the lessons it offers.
I want to know why I carry this affliction
so that I may rid myself of its grasp on my body.

DAY 9

Thought for the Day
SELF-ANALYSIS

Affirmation

I am now on the path of healing.
I listen to the messages that my body offers.
I listen to my wonderings.
I ask my body why am I carrying this affliction.
I search for answers within and outside of myself.

DAY 10

Thought for the Day
SIGNALS TO CHANGE

Affirmation

I am now on the path of healing.
I listen to the messages that my body offers.

I am observant.
I look for the signs of change that I need to undertake
in order to be healed.

DAY 11

Thought for the Day
SELF-EFFORT

Affirmation

I am now on the path of healing.
I listen to the messages that my body offers.

I ask myself
'Am I doing everything possible to facilitate self-healing?'.

DAY 12

Thought for the Day
SELF-ANALYSIS

Affirmation

I am now on the path of healing.
I listen to the messages that my body offers.

I examine myself to ensure I am doing
everything possible to facilitate self-healing.

DAY 13

Thought for the Day
SELF-EFFORT

Affirmation

I am now on the path of healing.
I listen to the messages that my body offers.

I seek to be doing everything possible
to facilitate self-healing.

DAY 14

Thought for the Day
CONTENTMENT

Affirmation

I am now on the path of healing.
I listen to the messages that my body offers.

I relax in knowing
I am doing everything possible to facilitate self-healing.

7
COMMONLY ASKED QUESTIONS

*E*NQUIRY IS part of the human psy-
che. People who are interested in my abilities will either ask
superficial questions or interrogate me. I always answer
truthfully and as simply as I can, since I know they seek re-
assurance. Every time a new client comes to me I am asked
five or more of the following questions. I am pleased to share
their enquiries with you to serve as a quick reference.

WHEN DID YOU REALISE YOU COULD HEAL PEOPLE?
After thinking long and hard, I realise I have been a healer all
my life. In some form or another I have brought peace to the
lives of others. However, one particular incident in my life
determined the awakening of my hands-on healing path
under spiritual guidance (see page 2).

WHERE DO YOU BELIEVE THE HEALING COMES FROM?
I believe it is Divine in nature. Its simple power suggests
Godliness.

DO YOU BELIEVE YOU HAVE BEEN BLESSED BY GOD?
I believe we are all blessed in different ways. Some of us
choose to recognise it and work while others ignore their
blessing and struggle with life.

HOW DOES THE HEALING WORK?
I act as a vessel that facilitates Divine intervention. When I place my hands above or on an ailment the healing automatically commences, supplied and directed by a Divine source.

DO YOU HAVE TO BELIEVE IN SPIRITUAL HEALING TO BE CURED?
I have learnt from experience that no faith is required in order to be healed.

DO YOU BELIEVE YOU CAN CURE EVERYONE?
No. I don't class myself as a miracle worker. I believe that if you are meant to be cured you will be. The healing comes from a Divine source, not me.

WHY DO SOME PEOPLE HEAL QUICKLY AND OTHERS MORE SLOWLY?
I believe that illness teaches a person a lot about themselves and also teaches an appreciation for life. We heal at the rate we are meant too.

WHAT IS MEANT BY SPONTANEOUS HEALING?
I have noticed that in the case of spontaneous healing, the physical, emotional and attitudinal symptoms cure at the same time, producing a collective and spontaneous release of illness.

CAN YOU PREDICT WHO WILL BE SPONTANEOUSLY HEALED?
I predict this only when I recognise that an ailment is drawing out the healing from me at a powerful rate.

HOW DO YOU KNOW HOW MANY HEALING SESSIONS THE TREATMENT OF AN AILMENT WILL TAKE?
I have learnt from experience. For example, if a migraine isn't cured in the first session, it will usually take up to five sessions to cure. Specific ailments have specific response times to healing.

DOES THE HEALING DRAIN YOU?

Not at all. I use my own energy to sit, stand and talk only. On the contrary, it usually takes me about one hour to regain my humanness after healing for nine hours per day.

I have to ground a sensation of floating.

DO YOU CONTINUALLY HAVE TO PROVE YOUR SKILLS?

Only to those who fall into the Doubting Thomas group and to the media, who I think are professional sceptics. Often it seems they are more interested in proving me wrong than right, while the 'doubters' are happy to be proved wrong.

WHO HEALS YOU?

Usually my husband Paul and sister-in-law Lorraine. He is an iridologist, a gifted Bowen practitioner and an aromatherapist. She is a very talented homoeopath. I also know some of the best doctors and dentists.

DOES ANY OTHER PERSON IN YOUR FAMILY SHARE YOUR GIFT?

My niece Carolan Nicholson has worked as my assistant for several years. I first recognised her ability when she was fifteen years old. My grandfather, who died when I was three years old, apparently had intuitive abilities.

IS IT A REWARDING EXPERIENCE?

Everyday I go home with a smile on my face because someone has been healed or relieved of pain. Everyday, the healing rewards me for my devotion.

WHAT DO YOU THINK OF DOCTORS?

I think they are like any other group of professional people. Some are more gifted than others and some are more enthusiastic workers than others.

WHAT DO DOCTORS THINK ABOUT WHAT YOU DO?

Like everyone else in the community, some believe in it and others don't. Everyone in a free world is entitled to their own opinion.

DO MANY PROFESSIONAL PEOPLE COME TO SEE YOU?
People from all walks of life are equal in cancer and the like.
I see not their profession, only their needs. I find everyone
fascinating to treat: the butcher, the baker and the candle-
stick maker. I love treating real estate agents because their
business is my hobby.

HOW DO RELIGIOUS GROUPS RESPOND TO YOU?
Countless ministers, priests and nuns have passed through
my clinic. I find their beliefs in keeping with my philosophy
of spiritual healing being Divine intervention.

ARE YOU A MIRACLE WORKER?
We are all miracles of life. My role is to be a vessel for energy
to give service to people through the power of Divine love.
The knowledge I bring to healing has been acquired from
experience of treatment over many years.

RECOMMENDED LISTENING

HERE IS a list of music which I highly recommend and which I use during healing sessions. The combined skills of the composer and the musicians help to lift the mind to a level of release, contemplation, self-exploration and healing.

Instrumental music for relaxation, meditation and self-healing
Asha: *Celestine* — tracks 1, 2, 3, 4, 8 and 10
Deep Forest: *Deep Forest* — tracks 9 and 10.
Kamal: *Into Silence* — all tracks.
Kitaro: *The Light of the Spirit* — tracks 1, 3 and 5.
Kitaro: *Tunhuang* — all tracks except 4 and 7.
Tony O'Connor: *Mariner* — all tracks.
Tony O'Connor: *Uluru* — tracks 1, 2, 4, 6 and 8.
Terry Oldfield: *Illumination* — all tracks.
Rainchild: *Trance-ition* — tracks 1, 2 and 6.
Vangelis: *Soil Festivities* — tracks 2 and 4.
Vangelis: *Portraits* — tracks 4, 10, 11 and 14.
Vangelis: *Voices* — tracks 4 and 9.

Instrumental music for family and friends healing circles
John Barry: *Out of Africa* (soundtrack) — all tracks except 6 and 10.
Peter Gabriel: *Birdy* — all tracks except 2, 7 and 9.
Vangelis: *L'Apocalypse des Animaux* — tracks 2, 4, 6 and 7.
Vangelis: *Direct* — tracks 4, 8, 9 and 11.
Vangelis: *Antarctica* — tracks 2, 5, 6 and 8.
Vangelis: *1492* — all tracks except 9 and 10.

Affirmative popular songs for emotional and mental self-healing
I have listed songs by popular artists who have either written or
recorded music which serves to deliver a personal message or
enhance your life, awakening new thinking patterns or reinforcing
your self-esteem and beliefs. You will notice that artists such as
Donovan and Bob Marley have devoted their musical career to
bringing hope and healing to their fellow man.

ARMSTRONG, Louis
'What a wonderful world'   Affirming the beauty of living.

THE CARS
'Good times roll'   Creating a positive reality.
'Shake it up'   Releasing tension and chaos.

COLD CHISEL
'You got nothing I want'   Reinforcing of independence.

COODER, Ry
'What came first'   Questioning spiritual beliefs.
'Get rhythm when   Uplifting when depressed.
  you've got the blues'

THE CORRS
'Someday'   Releasing a relationship.

CROWDED HOUSE
'Instinct'   Attuning to your intuition.
'Everything is good for you'   Reinforcing your life.

DONOVAN
'Only the blues'   Releasing negative feelings.
'Happiness runs'   Reinforcing a positive reality.
'The sun is a very magic fellow'   Consolidating an affinity with
                                        nature.
'Someone's singing'   Reinforcing personal happiness.
'Maya's dance'   Spiritual awakening.
'Wear your love like heaven'   Spiritual self-reflection.
'What the soul desires'   Giving the soul a voice for self-
                                        expression.
'The mountain'   Assessing one's place in the world.

'Harmony'	Creating balance of mind, body and soul.
'The great song of the sky'	Reinforcing a peaceful community spirit.
'There is an ocean'	Attuning to your mind and soul.
'Deathless delight'	Attuning to the spirit body.
'Sailing homeward'	Positively releasing the body to death.
Sutras (album)	Personal enlightenment.

THE DOORS

'Been down so long'	Getting out of a self-destructive rut.

EURYTHMICS

'Sweet dreams'	Strengthening personal character.
'Right by your side'	Attracting True Love.
'There must be an angel'	Spiritual awareness and enhancement.
'When tomorrow comes'	Coping with a turbulent relationship.
'Miracle of love'	Comforting during emotional devastation.

FLEETWOOD MAC

'Don't stop'	Overcoming a poor reality.
'Go your own way'	Releasing a relationship amicably.
'My little demon'	Helping to identify and release negative attitudes.

GERRY AND THE PACEMAKERS

'You'll never walk alone'	Encouraging strength to cope with trials.

GERSHWIN, George (composer)
(sung by numerous popular artists)

'Nice work if you can get it'	Attracting a relationship.
'I'll build a stairway to paradise'	Motivating success in life.

JOEL, Billy

'River of dreams'	Encouraging awareness of the dream/Spirit world.

KING, Carole
'Tapestry'   Positive self-reflection on life.
'You've got a friend'   Reinforcing the values of a relation-
                                    ship.

KNOPFLER, Mark
'Nobody's got the gun'   Encouraging the sharing of responsi-
                                    bility in a relationship.
'I'm the fool'   Overcoming mistakes in a relation-
                                    ship.

LED ZEPPELIN
'Stairway to heaven'   Spiritual guidance.

LITTLE RIVER BAND
'Shut down, turn off'   Letting go of daily hassles in prepa-
                                    ration for sleep.
'Curiosity killed the cat'   Overcoming negative attitude
                                    towards love.
'Lonesome loser'   Overcoming the challenges of life.
'Help is on its way'   Re-evaluating attitude and lifestyle.
'My own way home'   Motivating for a better sense of
                                    direction.

McCARTNEY, Paul
'Hope of deliverance'   Releasing a sense of hopelessness.
'Somebody cares'   Releasing a sense of being alone.
'Calico skies'   Reaffirming the bond of a loving
                                    relationship.

McGOVERN, Maureen
'When you wish upon a star'   Creating a positive reality.
'Over the rainbow'   Creating hope.
'Swinging on a star'   Motivating for personal improve-
                                    ment.

McGRAW, Tim
'Wouldn't want it any other way'   Overcoming hard times and the tests
                                    of a relationship.
'Not a moment too soon'   Being thankful for receiving love
                                    and support.

McKENNITT, Loreena
'Dark night of the soul'   Spiritual soul searching.
'Full circle'   Spiritual soul searching.

McLEAN, Don
'It's a beautiful world'   Reinforcing a positive reality.
'Someone to watch over me'   Attracting a relationship.
'Count your blessings'   Reinforcing a positive reality.

MARLEY, Bob
'Three little birds'   Creating a positive reality.
'One love'   Affirming world peace.
'Satisfy my soul'   Creating balance in relationships.

MOODY BLUES
Threshold of a Dream (album)   Reinforcing personal strength and
                                  spirituality.

MOVING PICTURES
'What about me'   Reinforcing strength of character
                                  and self-identity.

MURRAY, Anne
'You needed me'   Reinforcing a caring relationship.

NELSON, Willie
'Blue skies'   Creating a positive reality.

O'SHEA, Mark
'World-weary heart'   Coming to terms with the stress of
                                  life.
'The dreamer'   Encouraging hope to succeed.

POLICE
'Spirits in the material world'   Spiritual awakening.

SIMON and GARFUNKEL
'I am a rock'   Reinforcing strength of character.
'Bookends theme'   Grieving loss.
'Song for the asking'   Reinforcing creativity and a positive
                                  reality.

STEVENS, Cat
'The wind'   Communicating with your soul.
'Tuesday's dead'   Changing your reality for the better.

10CC
'Life is a minestrone'   Sorting out issues in life positively.
'Wall street shuffle'   Creating abundance.
'Things we do for love'   Assessing patterns in a relationship.

VAN ZALM, Peggy
'Soul magic'   Opening yourself to your soul.
'Parallel journeys'   Seeking unconditional love.
'Spiral dancing'   Awakening the rhythm of the soul.

RECOMMENDED READING

Healing diet

Bobbin, T. & Horne, R. 1984, *Anti-Cancer, Anti-Heart Attack Cookbook*, Happy Landings, Sydney.

Cabot, Dr Sandra 1996, *The Liver Cleansing Diet*, WHAS, Sydney.

Jameson, Judy 1994, *Fat-Burning Foods*, Ottenheimer, USA.

Marsden, Kathryn 1994, *Food Combiner's Meal Planner*, Thornsons, London.

Murray, Dr Michael T. 1992, *The Complete Book of Juicing*, Prima Publishing,

Pentecost, Marlene 1985, *Cooking for your Life*, Reed Books, Sydney.

Porter, Suzanne 1985, *It's Only Natural*, Greenhouse, Melbourne.

Porter, Suzanne 1986, *Simply Healthy*, Greenhouse, Melbourne.

Porter, Suzanne 1989, *Keeping it Low with Meat*, self-published.

Pritikin, Nathan 1985, *The Pritikin Promise*, Bantam Books, New York.

Samways, Louise 1989, *The Chemical Connection*, Greenhouse, Melbourne.

Schaeffer, Severen L. 1987, *Instinctive Nutrition*, Celestial Arts, Berkeley.

Stafford, Julie 1984, *Taste of Life*, Greenhouse, Melbourne.

Stafford, Julie 1985, *More Taste for Life*, Greenhouse, Melbourne.

Stafford, Julie 1989, *Conquering Cholesterol*, Greenhouse, Melbourne.

Stafford, Julie 1994, *Juicing for Health*, Viking, Melbourne.

Organic gardening

Collins, Judith 1993, *Companion Gardening in Australia*, Lothian, Melbourne.

Dean, Esther 1977, *Gardening — Growing without Digging*, Harper &
Row, Sydney.
Morrow, Rosemary 1993, *Earth Users Guide to Permaculture*,
Kangaroo Press, Kenthurst.

Self-empowerment
Collins, Judith 1997, *Affirmations for Life*, Lothian, Melbourne.
Jackson, Dr Gary 1997, *Brain Food*, self-published (available from G.
Jackson, 140 Newburn Road, High Wycombe, WA 6057,
Telephone/Fax: (08) 9454 3661.

Cancer and heart disease
Cilento, Dr Ruth 1993, *Heal Cancer*, Hill of Content, Melbourne.
Quillin, Dr Patrick 1994, *Beating Cancer with Nutrition*, Nutrition
Times Press, Tulsa.

Spirituality
Collins, Judith 1993, *Beads of Wisdom*, Canticle Productions, Picton.
Vine, Rosalie 1996, *Other Ways of Knowing*, Comet Communications,
Campbelltown.
Vine, Rosalie 1998, *Other Ways of Being*, Comet Communications,
Campbelltown.

Meditation, relaxation and stress management
Collins, Judith, audio cassette recordings.
Collins, Judith 1994, *The Gift of Healing*, Canticle Productions,
Picton.
Collins, Judith 1994, *Meditative Journeys*, vols 1 & 2, Canticle
Productions, Picton.
Collins, Judith 1996, *Stress Relief*, Canticle Productions, Picton.

Other
Birdsall, George, *Feng Shui*, Advisory Centre, PO Box 278, Spit
Junction, NSW 2088.
Worwood, Valerie Ann 1994, *The Fragrant Pharmacy*, Bantam Books,
London.

USEFUL ADDRESSES

Judith Collins
Earthkeepers Healing Sanctuary
Coordinates Judith's private consultations and courses.
45 Addison Street
THIRLMERE, NSW 2572
Tel: (02) 4681 8543, Fax: (02) 4681 8280

Canticle Productions
For Judith's meditation and healing tapes and literature.
PO Box 163
PICTON, NSW 2571
Tel: (02) 4681 8543

Australian Traditional Medicine Society (ATMS)
Unit 12/27 Bank Street
MEADOWBANK, NSW 2114
Tel: (02) 9809 6800, Fax: (02) 9809 7570

Association of Remedial Masseurs (ARMS)
PO Box 440
RYDE, NSW 2112
Tel: (02) 9807 4769, Fax: (02) 9807 4454

Natural Health Society of Australia
Suite 28, 8 Skiptons Arcade
541 High Street
PENRITH, NSW 2750
Tel: (02) 4721 5068

National Herbal Society
PO Box 61
BROADWAY, NSW 2007
Tel: (02) 9211 6437, Fax: (02) 9211 6452

The Register of Acupuncture
31 Ada Place
ULTIMO, NSW 2007
Tel: (02) 9660 7708

Chinese Medicine & Herbal Centre of Sydney
392 Sussex Street
SYDNEY, NSW   2000
Tel: (02) 9261 8863, Fax: (02) 9261 2828

NEW ZEALAND
Spiritualist Church of New Zealand
40 Hautana Street
PO Box 45083
LOWER HUTT
NEW ZEALAND 6315
Tel: (04) 567 4085, Fax: (04) 567 4094

ASTROLOGERS
Private and mail order consultations.

Dawn Clark
2 Kalang Road
KENTHURST, NSW 2156
Tel: (02) 9654 2730

Paul Collins
PO Box 163
PICTON, NSW 2571
Tel: (02) 4681 9623
Tel: (02) 4681 8280